IT DOESN'T GET ANY

STRAIGHT-FORWARD INFORMATION THAT CAN CHANGE YOUR LIFE

Love you, Terry
— Mary

1
THING
"diet"

A LEADING AUTHORITY IN THE FIELDS OF OBESITY & DIABETES AT YALE UNIVERSITY

Mary Savoye-DeSanti, RD, CD-N, CDE

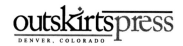

outskirtspress
DENVER, COLORADO

1 Thing "diet"
It Doesn't Get Any Simpler....Straight-Forward Information That Can Change Your Life
All Rights Reserved.
Copyright © 2012 Mary Savoye-DeSanti, RD, CD-N, CDE
v4.0

Cover design by Harrison Tonne of Rapture Image, LLC.

Visit our website at 1thingdiet.com

10% of all proceeds of this book will be donated to the American Diabetes Association and obesity and diabetes programs at the Pediatric Endocrinology Department of Yale University School of Medicine.

Outskirts Press, Inc.
http://www.outskirtspress.com

ISBN: 978-1-4327-8191-0

Library of Congress Control Number: 2012900192

Outskirts Press and the "OP" logo are trademarks belonging to Outskirts Press, Inc.

PRINTED IN THE UNITED STATES OF AMERICA

This book is dedicated to my beloved mother and father
who have instilled a hard work ethic in me and taught me—simply by my watching—to
reach out to others whenever possible.

It is also dedicated to all of the patients and families I have counseled over the years.
We have taught each other and passed our knowledge and experience on to
those needing similar support.

Table of Contents

Acknowledgements

I am deeply grateful for the patience and love of my family: My husband, Joseph DeSanti, sons, Michael and Cameron DeSanti, and daughter, Kaye Thomasina DeSanti. I would also like to acknowledge the love and support of other family and friends such as Teresa and Gary Preziosi, Tony DeLucia, Domenic and Domenique DeLucia, Paola and Brad Serrecchia, Lindsey Ertel, Jocelyn and Harrison Tonne, Carlton Savoye, Cindy Gonzalez, Jackie Cascio, Enit Colon, Michelle Morley, Beth Cusano, Hajra Jaffer, and Gina Barbetta.

I work or have worked with talented, loving colleagues and friends who have shown support, and in some cases reviewed my manuscript; these people include Melissa Shaw, Sonia Caprio, Bill Tamborlane, Katie Marotto, Patty Gatcomb, Sylvia Lavietes, Paulina Rose, Cindy Guandalini, Alisa Scherban, Grace Kim, Bridget Pierpont, Rachel Goldberg-Gell, Miladys Palau Collazo, Kerry Stephenson, Bob Sherwin, Rosa Hendler, and Paulina Nowicka. I express a special thanks to Paulina Nowicka who gave the book its name.

Many of my family members and friends have believed in me over the years more than I have believed in myself. I thank God for being surrounded by them. I also thank God for all the patients I have counseled over the years. Knowing and encouraging each and every one of them has truly been a blessing.

Introduction

I waited a long time to write this book because I thought what I had to say about weight loss was simply common sense and lacked a gimmick. Let's face it, most diet books have some kind of gimmick or plan to them that you must follow to see results. This is not a diet book, however. It is an opinion based on over twenty years of professional experience—most as dietitian and researcher—in the fields of obesity and diabetes and years of personal experience dieting while in my late teens and early twenties.

The decision to write this book was also ignited by the tremendous increase in the prevalence of type 2 diabetes. As the problem of obesity increases, so does type 2 diabetes. Unlike obesity, the development of diabetes is not considered a "cosmetic" problem anymore. Diabetes is a serious threat to one's health. Overweight individuals are at risk of developing diabetes.

This book is about as easy as it gets. My premise involves making one, hardly-noticeable change in your lifestyle every day. Diets come and go, they require far too much effort and, quite frankly, do not teach an overweight person any life skills to improve their weight problem long-term. I refer to diets as putting a bandage on the problem. Diets temporarily solve the problem. Why temporarily? If you cannot continue with "the plan," the change never becomes permanent and you, consequently, do not reap the benefits of it. I hope you will appreciate straightforward, fairly-simple information that can change your life permanently.

My beloved dad once said to me, "Perfectionists never get anything done." He was right. If something needs to be done perfectly, it takes the perfectionist forever to do their task. I have been tweaking this book for years and the truth is: It's time to get it out to the public. So while it's not perfect, it does contain valuable information that I believe will help anyone trying to lose weight and, consequently, improve their health.

PART ONE:

Reality Check (Attitude)

CHAPTER 1:

One Thing (Change) Means a Lot

If you are reading this book, you are most likely overweight or there is someone rather special in your life who is overweight. You are about to learn straightforward facts and examples, because, as stated earlier, I don't have a gimmick, a magic pill, or a special diet plan. While I can't promise you or your loved one that pounds will melt within 48 hours, I can promise you that you will learn some eye-opening facts about diet, behavior change, and weight loss that will stay with you forever.

Food has calories. We need calories for energy (energy to walk or get out of bed in the morning, for that matter). Food also has nutrients. Nutrients are vitamins or minerals that help the body with special functions (such as helping your heart pump, keeping your skin healthy…). You can get little nutrients for your calories or you can get a lot of nutrients for your calories (sort of like you can get a lot for your money or a little). The trick is to learn how to get the most nutrients in the fewest calories. This keeps you healthy while keeping your weight in check.

The chapter on "Nutrition 101 and Donuts 540" covers this whole concept of the nutrient value of food in more detail. I want to tell you about the little changes people have made in their diet simply by knowing the differences in values and having the guts or determination to put this knowledge into action.

A man I know named Peter took the train into New York from Connecticut every weekday. He read the daily newspaper and caught up on his work while making his commute. Like popcorn goes with watching a movie, this man would eat peanuts every day while reading the paper during his commute. He had this habit for quite a while and then, after learning that pretzels were lower in fat and calories, decided to switch from peanuts to pretzels. Within one year, this man lost 17 pounds! While there was only a difference of about 100 calories between the peanuts and pretzels, it was enough to make a difference five days a week for a year.

A patient of mine named Beverly came to see me several years ago. There was a lot of room for improvement in her diet. She enjoyed fast food restaurants and had a bit of a sweet tooth. What stood out to me, however, was that she drank three cans of cola a day. There was disbelief on her face when I told her that the only change I was suggesting was to give up the regular soda and switch to diet soda. "You're kidding, right?" she said to me. "You're not going to give me a diet plan to follow?" After switching to a diet cola and Fresca, this woman lost 14 pounds in three months!

Many times, it requires only one small change we apply every day to get results. If I had suggested five other changes along with this change in beverage, Beverly most likely would have had a hard time making all of these changes, reverted to old behaviors and, consequently, made no progress at all.

It takes only 3500 excess calories consumed to equal one pound of body fat. That means, every 3500 extra calories consumed will cause a one-pound weight gain. To show you how easily calories add up, let's consider a teaspoon of sugar—yes, one itty, bitty teaspoon of sugar that has only 15 calories. If you were to put two teaspoons of sugar in your coffee every day and you had already consumed your caloric needs for the day, you would gain over two pounds in one 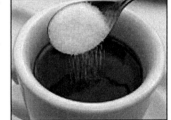 year. If you had two cups of coffee each day, it would develop into a 4 ½ pound weight gain by the end of the year. If you drank an 8-ounce glass of orange juice each day for breakfast instead of a 12-ounce glass, by the end of the year you would save about 21,900 calories or 6 ¼ pounds! Not bad for cutting back a bit! I think you get my point by now.

Also, one change in activity leads to calories burned and, therefore, weight loss. The chapter entitled "Get Up Off the Sofa!" gives you specific ideas about how to increase your activity level in a reasonable way. My favorite story regarding the effects of daily activity, however, is of Mrs. Cunningham, a quiet, conservative 62-year old woman. I used to work at a weight loss center in my heyday. This program consisted of packaged foods and lifestyle changes. Mrs. Cunningham claimed to be following the food plan faithfully every day with an occasional treat here and there. She would come in to the center for her weekly weigh-ins with great hope only to find a modest weight loss or no weight loss at all.

As a counselor, I would broach the subject of exercise very cautiously. Mrs. Cunningham never participated in formal exercise in her life. She was extremely sedentary. She enjoyed bridge and playing the piano, but never took part in physical activity. Each week I would bring up the subject of activity. She had many excuses—from lacking the right shoes to wear for exercise to getting leg cramps. I think her excuses were actually fears. She was afraid of doing something that was so foreign to her. My suggestions would get easier and easier as the weeks and months passed. I finally asked her if she thought she could walk to her mailbox each day. She had a fairly long driveway so she generally picked the mail up in her car as driving by each day. She laughed at my suggestion and quietly said, "I guess so," but I didn't take her seriously at all. In fact, it wasn't until several weeks later that I noticed Mrs. Cunningham was consistently losing a pound a week. I turned to her and asked if she was exercising and she just smiled at me. This woman lost twenty pounds once exercise became part of her daily regimen.

I worked as a dietitian at a community health center where I met a man David in his early 50s who had diabetes and high blood pressure. David was on Diabeta, a pill to control blood sugar. His blood pressure was elevated at 150/90 mmHg (target for adults with diabetes is less than 130/80 mmHg). David lost weight for two reasons: he started eating vegetables (something he never ate as a child or an adult) and he "found exercise." His car broke down one day while driving to work and, consequently, he started walking to his job. His funds were low so fixing his car right away was out of the question. He decided to walk to work the next day, too. Luckily his job was local (about two miles from his home), but it was certainly a workout for him. He would walk to work and hitch a ride home from a co-worker. While his car was inoperable, he walked to the grocery store and did other errands by foot (even our appointments!). My point is, he started to get more exercise than he ever got in his adult life! He is an extreme example here, but David made only one change in diet: adding string beans and carrots, the rest was solely (I couldn't resist!) walking.

Oh, I forgot to tell you the best part from a medical perspective: David's blood sugar became normal and he was able to discontinue the diabetes medication. His blood pressure also returned to normal. This man lost 21 pounds—or about 10% of his body weight—and it changed his life tremendously.

I have seen similar situations with children, as well. I started a weight management program for children at Yale several years ago. Shortly after, however, I started to offer a diabetes education class for children with type 2 diabetes that primarily focuses on weight loss for children with diabetes to improve their blood sugar control. The program encourages parents or care givers to attend the classes with their children. A patient I am particularly proud of is Monica, a 12-year-old girl (young woman now) with type 2 diabetes, who was on both Glucophage (an oral medication for diabetes) and insulin. After ten months, Monica lost 21 pounds and was able to discontinue all medication, including the insulin. The change Monica made was actually a family change. Her mom did not buy any more of the following junk foods: ice cream, cookies, and chips. Mom also bought Monica Crystal Light (a sugar-free, one-calorie drink), which the family also started to drink right along with her instead of Kool-aid. Sugar-free gelatin with cool whip took the place of ice cream, fresh fruit took the place of cookies, and pretzels and air-popped popcorn took the place of chips.

In the same way that we do not need to make big changes in our diet or activity level to see weight loss results, we often do not need to lose a lot of weight to see health benefits. A 10-pound weight loss can help manage your high blood pressure. A 20-pound weight loss may help you come off the medication for type 2 diabetes. We have been brainwashed to believe that we have to reach our "ideal body weight" to become healthy. Nonsense! A modest weight loss can make the difference between going on medication or not. Incidentally, the term "ideal body weight" doesn't exist anymore. Not only did it have a Barbie-doll tone to it, the values were based on an outdated insurance table which was developed by self-reported weights. Since people rarely admit to their actual weight, typical weights of individuals were grossly understated. The term has been changed many times over. From "ideal" it went to "desirable" which wasn't much better. Then the term "realistic" took its place. Now the preferred phrase is "healthy" body weight, which is a term defined as the weight at which you and your doctor (I say dietitian!) feel you can realistically maintain and that which brings health benefits.

But back to real health results from diet changes: Several studies exist that show similar results to what I am presenting (some people like to see the scientific evidence!). I'm not referring to new information. These studies have been around for a while. In fact, I will show you older studies just to prove that the concept of modest weight loss to achieve improved health has been around for a long time. One study, dating back to 1987, published in the Archives of Internal Medicine (Wing R, 1987), showed that just a 15-pound weight loss after one year resulted in a significant improvement in blood sugar (indicated by a hemoglobin A1% or HgA1% drop).

HgA1% Before and After Weight Loss

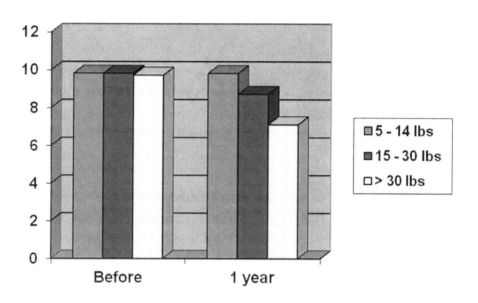

Wing R, Arch Intern Med, 1987

A hemoglobin A1 is part of the hemoglobin or red blood cell that can be measured to see how much of the sugar in the blood actually attached itself to the red blood cell (the higher the percentage, the more damage or attachment). Currently, hemoglobin A1c percentages are most commonly used by the medical profession to determine blood sugar control. They are a smaller area of the red blood cell than the HgA1 and measure control over the last 90 days, the life span of the red blood cell and typically the time between follow-up clinic appointments.

This study showed a drop from 9.8% HgA1 to 8.7% HgA1 after such a modest loss (15 to 30 pounds). Why am I emphasizing the group that lost 15 to 30 pounds and not the group that lost the most? Because I want to remain realistic and promote the concept of moderate, achievable goals. It's not about winning a gold medal, it's about reaching a little bit further than you normally would, even if that means just getting your walking shoes or sneakers on and walking around the block. Bottom line about diabetes management is that each one percent drop means less heart, eye, kidney, and nerve disease. There has been a landmark study called the Diabetes Control and Complications Trial or DCCT which clearly found that a 1.5% drop in HgA1c equated to a 41 to 76 % decrease in risk of the above-mentioned complications.

Similar results are seen when weight loss results in improvements in blood pressure (again, these studies are not new). High blood pressure or hypertension is an elevation of the pressure of blood flow in a person's arteries. This is the most common disease of the heart and blood vessels. The top number is called the systolic blood pressure, while the bottom number is referred to as the diastolic blood pressure. Systolic BP is the peak pressure when the *heart contracts* as it pumps blood *out* of the heart. Diastolic BP is the pressure when the *heart relaxes* to permit the *inflow* of blood.

While the definition for high blood pressure is >140/90 mmHg, the target is actually lower for individuals with diabetes since high blood pressure can be more problematic for this population. The American Diabetes Association and the National Institute of Health recommend a blood pressure <130/80 mmHg for adults with diabetes.

Almost two out of every four adult Americans are afflicted with high blood pressure and it is twice as common among individuals with diabetes as in the general population. African Americans are also more likely to have high blood pressure than the general population. Having hypertension with diabetes is part of a syndrome or cluster of disorders called the Metabolic Syndrome.

In 1997 Agurs-Collins and colleagues did a short-term study to measure improvements in both glucose and blood pressure in African Americans with type 2 diabetes. What I really like about this study was that the subjects lost only 5 pounds in a 3- to 6-month period. The study showed the following results:

- 1 to 2.4% drop in HgA1c (measures blood sugar control)
- drop of 4 mmHg diastolic blood pressure
- drop of 8.4 mmHg systolic blood pressure
  Agurs-Collins TD, et al, Diabetes Care, 1997

To sum things up, modest weight loss can change one's health significantly. And how do you achieve a modest weight loss? Make one change in your lifestyle that is contributing to your weight problem. In other words, choose "1 thing" that you honestly believe will make a difference. It's perhaps too soon to know what *your* "1 thing" will be. You most likely need to learn more about yourself, including your attitude, which I'll cover in the next chapter. However, before I end this chapter, would you like to know if David ever got his car fixed? Yes, he did. We'll go back to David in a later chapter.

CHAPTER 2:

Get Real!—Why Crash Diets Don't Work!

The Scene: A donut shop one block from my house.

I run into my cousin, Charlie, who looks at me strangely while I am checking out at the register.

Charlie: Hi Mary, I thought you lost so much weight (he heard this from family members).

Mary: I did, I just gained it back already.

He offered to pay for my donuts. I smiled nicely and declined out of pure embarrassment.

My years of experience have shown that it is hard for people to be realistic with their weight loss expectations. They want to lose the weight and they want to lose it now! This is understandable, although very unrealistic. Who doesn't want a quick weight loss? Who in their right mind wants to work hard at weight loss? We want to do the least and get the most for our efforts. Well, in some ways, this book is about doing the least for the most. If you really don't want to work hard, this is the book for you. But let's take a look at how unrealistic—and unhealthy—some of our wishes are.

Do you think it's realistic for a 50-year-old man to weigh the same as he did in high school? Do you think it's realistic for a 45-year-old woman to weigh the same weight as the day she married her second husband 16 years ago? I hope you answered NO to both of these scenarios.

As the body ages, the metabolism slows down. Why? Because generally we lose muscle as we age. Muscle is more active in the body than fat is. Muscle burns calories four times faster than fat. The higher our percentage of muscle, the higher our metabolic rate (the rate at which we burn calories) or metabolism is. And, you guessed it, the higher our percent fat, the lower our metabolic rate or metabolism is.

Interestingly enough, when we crash diet, we lose weight quickly. The weight we are losing, however, is primarily muscle and water. It is a shame to lose precious muscle weight just to see the number on the scale go in a desired direction. The water comes back eventually, but the muscle is hard to recoup. It's a vicious cycle actually: when you crash diet, you lose muscle. When you lose muscle, your body is less efficient at burning calories (remember, fat only uses 25 percent the amount of calories that muscle uses!). What happens when the crash diet is over? You gradually gain weight back (oops, mostly fat, too). Now you have decreased your muscle and increased your fat, slowing down your metabolic rate. This explains why you often put more weight on after a crash diet because you go back to taking in the same number of calories as before, but the body is no longer burning calories as efficiently as before. So overall, crash dieting changes your muscle to fat ratio for the worse. When the fat is favored in this ratio, it is very hard to lose weight.

In addition to losing muscle, crash dieting causes diuresis (loss of water in the body). Water weighs a lot. Have you ever weighed a glass of water? Eight ounces of water weighs ¾ of a pound. Yes, almost a pound! It is worth noting that the "low carbohydrate craze" promotes water loss. You may be wondering why a low carbohydrate diet brings on water loss. If so, let me explain this in a simple way.

When you eat carbohydrates, they turn into glucose (sugar) in the body. If this glucose is not needed right away for energy, the glucose gets stored in the body as glycogen (stored energy). Glycogen can be thought of as glucose molecules stuck together. Glycogen is very necessary for quick energy. When we do not eat enough carbohydrate, our blood sugar drops. In order to bring the blood sugar back up, the body searches for glucose.

If there is no glucose in the blood from a recently consumed carbohydrate source, the body turns to its glycogen stores (stored glucose). With each release of glucose molecule from the glycogen, comes water. Picture knocking on the Glycogen residence door and saying "Can Glucose come out and play?" In this case, the parent would say, "Sure, but take his baby brother, Water, with you!" Glycogen and water travel together. When you tap into your glycogen stores, you automatically lose water. And if you are not eating much carbohydrate, you don't need the water that gets stored with the glucose. Both scenarios—using up stored carbohydrate or taking in less carbohydrate—mean less water and therefore, less weight when you step on the scale.

As you are most likely beginning to understand, the number on the scale doesn't tell the whole story. Body weight, per se, is a poor indicator of the percentage of body fat. It is important to know how much fat and muscle you have. Muscle, fat, and water primarily make up body weight (bone is a major component of body weight as well). Two people can weigh exactly the same and one can be overweight while the other is quite lean.

When I was nineteen years old, I was surprised to learn that I weighed nearly the same weight as my very lean friend, Wendy. When Wendy told me she weighed about 155 pounds, too, I was in shock: How could this be? She was thin! (Wendy was also taller than my 5' 3 ½" frame). Now I understand that she had much more muscle than I did. She had never dieted before either, while I was on my 86th diet—each time losing more and more muscle, I am sure.

There are many different ways to determine your body composition or how much muscle and fat you have. Products on the market referred to as body fat analyzers estimate the percentage of fat in the body. These are getting popular at health clubs and for home use. They are typically scale-like devices that have metal footpads to stand on. A small current runs through the body and crudely measures the amount of water in the body. Muscle likes water, fat doesn't. The higher the water reading, the higher the muscle reading. Most products are also scales. Some give a printout of weight and fat percentage among other values. These products are rough estimates and should be used for looking at trends only (is the percent body fat consistently going up or down, for example).

There are much more sophisticated and accurate techniques, but these are not practical for home use. Such highly-respected techniques include dual ex-ray absorptiometry (DEXA) and magnetic resonance imaging (MRI) and are mandatory in the research field because these tools offer highly accurate measurements of body fat and lean muscle.

If you use a body fat analyzer at home or at the gym, don't get hung up on an "ideal" percentage if it offers such information. Simply try to go in the right direction. Look for trends when you measure your percent body fat. If your body fat was 43% in January and then you check it again in March and it's 38%, this is great progress!

Women have a higher percentage of fat in their bodies than men (I tell you, it is such a man's world!). In general, women should be less than 35 percent fat and men should be less than 25 percent fat. Women need more adipose tissue (fat) on their bodies for reproductive reasons. Since females have a higher percentage of fat in their body than males, this tells us that it is easier for a man to lose weight than it is for a woman (remember, fat is less metabolically active than muscle). I have a hard time watching these weight loss competition shows on television when men are in the same category as women because it is so physically—and scientifically—unfair.

Speaking of unfair: I wonder what Barbie's percent body fat is. Did you know that if Barbie were a real person, she would have to remove her lowest rib in order for her to have such a small waist in proportion to her hips (no thank you, I'll keep my twelfth rib, please!). You know the old saying, "If something seems too good to be true…" The last I heard of Barbie, the feminists were recommending that you wrap elastic bands around her waistline before giving them to your precocious daughters so that the dolls would appear wider or more realistic (this is no joke!).

Moral of the story: be patient with weight loss. Lose slowly so you can lose fat, not water or precious muscle. Moreover, shoot for a realistic weight. A realistic weight can make the difference between success and failure. If your body cannot maintain a certain weight because it is physically impossible, why set yourself up to feel like you've failed miserably. If the weight you are striving for is not maintainable after diligently eating healthier and exercising regularly, it is probably not a good weight for you. Embrace your lower weight and congratulate yourself on your success.

The other moral of the story: Don't crash diet. In fact, don't diet at all. I truly believe that when we diet, we set ourselves up to feel deprived. This, in addition to losing muscle when we lose weight too fast, is a bad mix. Think about the last time you dieted. How did you feel? Did you keep the weight off?

Eleven years ago, I developed a weight management program for children at Yale. It's a wonderful program that has both national and international recognition. Why so much recognition? We see positive, long-term results. When I first developed the program, I felt strongly about the members *not* dieting. Let me tell you why. I dieted between ages sixteen and twenty-three and only gained weight as a long-term result. I tried every single diet on the market: The Scarsdale Diet (Now I'm really dating myself), the Diet Center, etc. It was not until I *stopped* dieting that I lost weight permanently.

Dieting sets people up for a black and white mentality—You are "off" or you are "on." When you're off, "it's a day at the races," as a dear obese 42-year old patient of mine has told me. When you're on, you have this belief that you have to eat only what is on the plan. Suddenly you want other foods; you might even start daydreaming about food. We need to find a balance here between "off to the races" and feeling like we are being punished.

To be sure that I was doing the right thing when I started a non-diet approach at the Yale Weight Management Program, Bright Bodies, I kept track of the kids using the non-diet philosophy and compared the results with kids who asked for something more structured (Savoye M, 2005). Let me clarify first that it was the parents who asked for something more structured because adults are from the "School of Dieting." Parents would walk up to me and say, "Mary, I need something more structured, I need something to follow." Because I aim to please (and would have lost the participation of the parent and child anyway), I decided to give the parent a meal plan for their child, which was their security blanket in the situation. They did not feel comfortable with the idea of not using a written meal plan. The meal plan was a very balanced one written by the American Dietetic Association. It was safe with adequate calories and nutrients, flexible with lots of choices, and very clear.

I followed this group for two years. Most kids used the suggested non-diet approach of making better food choices (popcorn v potato chips, for example) and eating moderate portion sizes (1 C pasta v 3 C, for example). At the end of the first year, I must say, I was a bit worried. The structured meal plan group (dieters) fared slightly better than the non-dieters. Wow, maybe I'm wrong, I thought. Perhaps all of the kids should be dieting?

Both groups lost weight and decreased their body mass index or BMI (see next chapter for explanation of BMI). Good news! I asked to see them again in one year (any good interventional study involves follow-up). Lo and behold, one year later (2-year mark), the dieters had gained all of their weight back, while the non-dieters continued to decrease their BMI. In fact, some dieters did not want to return to get reweighed because of shame. Of course, there was absolutely nothing for them to be ashamed of. They used the traditional—but wrong—method.

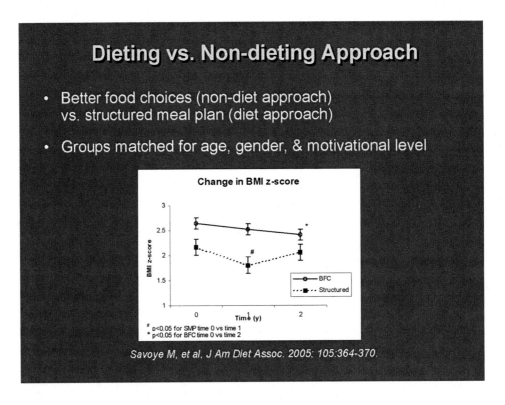

The saddest thing about these kids gaining the weight back is that they worked so hard, I am sure. The non-dieters also worked hard, but didn't beat themselves up as much and went about living their life in a regular way. The non-dieters still ate at parties, walked through the cafeteria line, ate pizza on Friday evenings. They just made conscious decisions about which food or how much they were about to eat. The dieters deprived themselves. The sooner we stop being so rigid with ourselves, the sooner we will lose weight and keep it off.

In summary—again—be patient with yourself, have realistic expectations, and don't be tempted to diet.

PART TWO:

Understanding Obesity and Diabetes (Background)

CHAPTER 3:

Obesity: What is it? How did it get here?

You can't change your genes, but you can change your jeans (size).
~~ Mary Savoye-DeSanti

There is not one culprit involved with being overweight. There's probably not two culprits either. While there may be several reasons for obesity, some causes remain poorly understood.

Before we get into the main reasons for obesity, I think a definition is called for. Obesity is defined as a body mass index of 30 or greater. What is a body mass index or BMI? It is a weight-to-height ratio that determines your degree of obesity and, consequently, how at risk you are for developing health-related complications.

If you like math, you might want to *calculate* your BMI. If math is not your strong point, go to the next paragraph. To calculate your BMI, divide your weight (in pounds) by 2.2. This gives your weight in kilograms. Now multiply your height in inches by 0.0254. This is your height in meters. Now multiply your height in meters by itself (we are squaring your height in meters). Finally, divide the answer of your weight calculation by the answer of your height calculation. The result is your BMI. The formula is as follows: BMI = weight (kg)/height (M^2).

If all of the above is too much of a rigamarole for you, simply look at the chart below. Find your height on the left and your weight on the top. Follow your weight down to the

BMI number listed. For example, let's say you are 5 feet, 3 inches tall or 63 inches tall or 160 cm and you weigh 185 pounds or 84.1 kg. Find 5'3" feet or 160 cm to the left and 185 pounds towards the top. Find the BMI at which this height and weight intersect. Your BMI is 32. This is in the "Obese" category. As stated earlier, a BMI of 30 or greater is defined as obese.

Body Mass Index (BMI) Chart

Weight	lbs	100	105	110	115	120	125	130	135	140	145	150	155	160	165	170	175	180	185	190	195	200	205	210	215
	kgs	45.5	47.7	50.0	52.2	54.5	56.8	59.1	61.4	63.6	65.9	68.2	70.5	72.7	75.0	77.3	79.5	81.8	84.1	86.4	88.6	90.9	93.2	95.5	97.7
Height	in/cm	Underweight						Healthy					Overweight					Obese					Morbidly obese		
5'0" -	152	19	20	21	22	23	24	25	26	27	28	29	30	31	32	33	34	35	36	37	38	39	40	41	42
5'1" -	155	18	19	20	21	22	23	24	25	26	27	28	29	30	31	32	33	34	35	36	36	37	38	39	40
5'2" -	157	18	19	20	21	22	22	23	24	25	26	27	28	29	30	31	32	33	33	34	35	36	37	38	39
5'3" -	160.0	17	18	19	20	21	22	23	24	24	25	26	27	28	29	30	31	32	32	33	34	35	36	37	38
5'4" -	163	17	18	18	19	20	21	22	23	24	24	25	26	27	28	29	30	31	31	32	33	34	35	36	37
5'5" -	165	16	17	18	19	20	20	21	22	23	24	25	25	26	27	28	29	30	30	31	32	33	34	35	35
5'6" -	168	16	17	17	18	19	20	21	21	22	23	24	25	25	26	27	28	29	29	30	31	32	33	34	34
5'7" -	170	15	16	17	18	18	19	20	21	22	22	23	24	25	25	26	27	28	29	29	30	31	32	33	33
5'8" -	172.7	15	16	16	17	18	19	19	20	21	22	22	23	24	25	25	26	27	28	28	29	30	31	32	32
5'9" -	175	14	15	16	17	17	18	19	20	20	21	22	22	23	24	25	25	26	27	28	28	29	30	31	31
5'10" -	178	14	15	15	16	17	18	18	19	20	20	21	22	23	23	24	25	25	26	27	28	28	29	30	30
5'11" -	180	14	14	15	16	16	17	18	18	19	20	21	21	22	23	23	24	25	25	26	27	28	28	29	30
6'0" -	183	13	14	14	15	16	17	17	18	19	19	20	21	21	22	23	23	24	25	25	26	27	27	28	29
6'1" -	158	13	13	14	15	15	16	17	17	18	19	19	20	21	21	22	23	23	24	25	25	26	27	27	28
6'2" -	188	12	13	14	14	15	16	16	17	18	18	19	19	20	21	21	22	23	23	24	25	25	26	27	27
6'3" -	191	12	13	13	14	15	15	16	16	17	18	18	19	20	20	21	21	22	23	23	24	25	25	26	26
6'4" -	193.0	12	12	13	14	14	15	15	16	17	17	18	19	19	20	20	21	22	22	23	23	24	25	25	26

A BMI of 30 equates to being approximately 30% above healthy weight and, of course, increases one's chance of having serious health problems associated with obesity, such as diabetes, heart disease, gallbladder disease, osteoarthritis, and specific cancers. A BMI of 27 equates to 20% above healthy weight. A BMI between 27 and 30 is defined as overweight. This definition of obesity and overweight using the BMI has gained more respect over the years as it clearly relates to health, unlike "ideal body weight" or "desirable body weight." Research shows that there is a relationship between BMI and mortality risk (Manson JE, 1995; Troiano R, 1996).

Shape Up America, a nonprofit organization whose mission includes combating obesity through education and treatment, have summarized an adult's health risk according to BMI as follows:

BMI Category	Health Risk
<25	minimal
25 - <27	low
27 - <30	moderate
30 - <35	high
35 - <40	very high
≥40	extremely high

It is worth noting that there is a major limitation to the use of BMI. BMI does not consider the amount of fat versus muscle of an individual. If you are an athlete or a body builder, BMI will not be a good assessment of obesity for you because of your high muscle mass. Also pregnant or lactating women should not use BMI. The use of BMI percentiles instead of simply a BMI number should be used to assess obesity in children. Children's BMI is age and gender specific, as they are still growing. Your child's pediatrician should be using a BMI percentile graph developed by the Center for Disease Control (CDC) if he or she is assessing their weight status.

Also a greater health risk is associated with centralized fat (abdominal area) versus gynoidal fat (hip and thigh area). Those who tend to carry fat in the upper body and abdomen area are referred to as "apple-shaped," while those who carry fat in the hips and thighs are referred to as "pear-shaped." It is riskier to be an apple-shaped overweight individual since the proximity of intra-abdominal fat to the major organs (heart, liver, for example) is apparent. Also, fat cells tend to be larger in the abdominal area and, therefore, have a higher rate of breakdown. When fat breaks down (lipolysis), free fatty acids are dispersed. These free fatty acids disrupt normal glucose metabolism or your body's ability to use glucose. It is not surprising to notice there are more apple-shaped individuals with Type 2 diabetes than pear-shaped individuals. We'll discuss this in a bit more detail in the next chapter, "Diabetes: The Wrath of Obesity."

In addition to BMI, a waist-to-hip ratio was developed to determine the health risk of obese individuals. The way to calculate the ratio is much easier than the BMI (I promise!). Simply measure your waist (approximately one inch above your belly button) in inches. This is W. Now measure your hips (the largest area is your true hip) in inches. This is H. Now divide W by H. For women, if your ratio is bigger than 0.8, you have centralized fat distribution (you are an apple!); if your ratio is less than 0.8, you have gynoidal fat distribution (you are a pear!). For men, if your ratio is larger than 1.0, you have centralized fat distribution (apple); if your ratio is less than 1.0, you have gynoidal fat distribution (pear). As stated earlier, it is riskier from a health standpoint to be apple-shaped.

Now getting back to the reasons for obesity. The two main reasons for obesity are *genetics* and *environment*. We know that obesity is *genetic*—that's right, inherited. You inherit your genes from your folks for eye color the same way that you inherit your genes for body weight. Did you ever notice how children are built like their mother or their father? Statistics exist regarding the chances of being overweight. If a child has one parent overweight, they have a 50% chance of being overweight. If both parents are overweight, his or her chances increase to 70%. Conversely, if neither parent is overweight, the child has a less than 10% chance of being overweight. Our metabolisms are genetically determined. We may think of our metabolism as the engine in our body. Some engines work very efficiently, while others are more sluggish.

Many of us clinicians hesitate to bear such daunting news of the genetic role in obesity because we are afraid of the response. We often hear "Well, what's the point in trying to lose weight if I've been genetically set to be fat?" What I tell my patients is this: "Yes, you are predisposed to obesity, but you can either sit back about it or try to minimize your weight gain." This is where *environment* comes into the picture.

Your environment is your home, your workplace, wherever you spend your time. Take a look around you now. Is your environment set up for being fit or being overweight? (I hate the F word in case you haven't noticed. I will hardly every say fat unless I am quoting a patient.) Is the television set turned on or are your children playing basketball outside? We are less active as a nation today than many years ago. We drive everywhere. We don't even get up to change the television or stereo channel. Many of us have a sedentary lifestyle or an environment that warrants little physical activity. What about our food intake? Ask yourself some of these questions: Did you prepare a balanced, home cooked meal or did you do take-out for dinner this evening? Is there a cookie jar or a fruit bowl on your counter? Is there ice cream in your freezer (who can ignore that at 9:00 p.m.)? We live in an environment today that conveniently offers high-fat food choices (entire books have been written on this unfortunate fact). Is your home a "safe" environment from a weight management perspective or is it loaded with temptations or eating triggers?

Dieting can be thought of as an environmental problem or contributor toward obesity. Your metabolism is genetically coded, but after years of dieting and changing your muscle to fat ratio, slowing down the metabolism more each time, we let the chronic habit of dieting sabotage our efforts very much like the familiar bag of chips in the cabinet.

These are all environmental factors that play a huge role in obesity. Let's face it, you have little control over genetics, but you have almost 100% control over your environment. We'll discuss this in greater detail in Chapter 12 (Becoming More Aware) and Chapter 13 (Taming of the Shrew: Making Those Necessary Changes).

In addition to genetics and environment, there are physical reasons we become overweight. One could argue that this is also genetic. A few examples are as follows: An overweight person that has high insulin levels might become more overweight. Insulin is a hormone (a product that circulates in the body and produces an effect on cells) created in the pancreas. It is an anabolic hormone. An anabolic hormone "builds" as opposed to breaking down. Insulin helps build tissue, it helps builds muscle and, yes, fat! Another example has to do with the newer hormone identified such as leptin. Leptin is a hormone made in the adipose (fat) tissue. Two things can go haywire with leptin. You can have a deficiency, although this is extremely rare, or you can have too much, which is more common. There are only a few cases of deficiency in the world and these people have been successfully treated with leptin injections (yes, they lost weight with leptin shots). Most people who have a problem with leptin, however, have a leptin resistance, which means that the leptin is not working efficiently because the cells are resistant to it. Anyway, these possible physical reasons of obesity are still in the experimental stages.

It is best to concentrate our weight loss efforts on what we know. We know that you can change your environment and lose weight with lifestyle changes. We also know that weight loss decreases all sorts of health problems. A major health problem associated with obesity (that inspired me to write this book) is diabetes.

CHAPTER 4

Diabetes: The Wrath of Obesity

Obesity and diabetes are "best friends."
~~ Dr. Sonia Caprio

Obesity and diabetes are "best friends," says Dr. Sonia Caprio, Professor of Pediatric Endocrinology at Yale University School of Medicine. She's right: They get along very well—in fact, too well. More than 90 percent of people with type 2 diabetes (the kind you generally get later in life and usually manage with a pill versus insulin) are overweight. With the increased prevalence of obesity and overall inactivity globally, it is estimated that the number of adults with diabetes will almost double by 2030 (Shaw J, 2010; Wild S, 2010). Of course aging and urbanization of society are also responsible for the diabetes surge, but the profound relationship between obesity and diabetes cannot be ignored.

This intense relationship between obesity and diabetes doesn't happen overnight. Diabetes takes years to develop. In fact, it is quite likely that you may be pre-diabetic for several years before you are actually diagnosed with full-blown diabetes.

For those of you who don't know what diabetes is, I will give you a description. When you have diabetes, you cannot use the sugar in your body normally. You eat food, it gets absorbed in the bloodstream, and instead of clearing within a certain amount of time, it builds up. There is a hormone made by the pancreas (an organ behind your stomach) called insulin that helps to keep your blood sugar levels normal. Glucose needs to get inside the cell for the cell to function properly, but it needs insulin to "let it in." Insulin is like a key to the lock. The lock can be considered a receptor (a fancy name for something that senses the presence of a particular hormone and latches on to it).

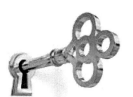

It wouldn't be a problem having all of this sugar build up in the blood but the darn sugar creates havoc for many of your tissues and organs. Picture the sugar molecules attaching themselves to necessary organs like your kidneys, heart, eyes, or nerves. Picture the sugar eating away at these tissues and damaging the organs over time. That's when you hear that Mrs. So and So had her leg amputated (sorry for the example).

Back to the job of the insulin keeping glucose in line. A major difference between type 1 diabetes and type 2 diabetes is that in type 1 the body doesn't have enough insulin (i.e., the pancreas doesn't make it), but in type 2 the body *does* makes insulin but it doesn't get used properly. In fact, the pancreas works overtime making extra insulin to keep blood sugars within normal levels. While it's working overtime, pre-diabetes (a condition in which blood sugar is between normal and diabetes) could be occurring, until eventually the pancreas can't keep up or even "burns out" and type 2 diabetes develops.

Obesity is responsible for changes that take place at the cell's surface (let's call these cell receptors that accept insulin). Picture a balloon getting blown up larger and larger. If you can imagine, the surface of the balloon would change. When the surface changes, the insulin receptors change, and the insulin does not recognize the receptor to latch on to. Result: Too much sugar or glucose in the blood, but interestingly enough, too much insulin in the blood as well (the insulin being made by the pancreas has nowhere to go either). In some cases, there are shortages of receptors on the level of the cell (different problem, but still a major difficulty if you're trying to clear glucose and insulin from the blood). The best analogy I have for a shortage of receptors or a problem with the receptors is what the parking lot looks like at the mall during the holidays—there are not enough parking spaces (receptors) for the cars (insulin). The horns blowing, etc. might symbolize the overflow of glucose in the blood.

There is a fundamental problem with obesity that leads to pre-diabetes or diabetes. This basic problem is that the body becomes *insulin resistant*. The body cannot use the insulin. When a person is overweight, there is generally an overflux of fatty acids in the blood. This is not only caused by too much fat in the blood from diet but also fat breaks down and builds up constantly. When it breaks down, fatty acids are the byproduct. These fatty acids are responsible for insulin resistance. They block the insulin from doing its job (poor insulin sensitivity).

With a lot of insulin in the blood (hyperinsulinemia), some people develop a skin condition known as acanthosis nigricans. Acanthosis, for short, is a darkening of the skin, particularly where there might be folds in the skin (neck, arm pits, groin, knuckles). In simple terms, the high levels of insulin in the blood go to the surface of the skin and change the pigmentation. A person with acanthosis most definitely is insulin resistant—maybe even pre-diabetic or has diabetes.

How would you know if you had pre-diabetes or diabetes, for that matter? A simple blood test can tell you if you have diabetes or one type of pre-diabetes called "impaired fasting glucose." If you have had nothing to eat after 10:00 p.m. the night before and the next morning and have your blood drawn in the morning (fasting) and your blood sugar is 126 or greater, this is considered diabetes. If your fasting blood sugar is between 100-125, you have "impaired fasting glucose" or pre-diabetes. If it is less than 100, your blood sugar is most likely normal. What do I mean, *most likely*…? Well, there is one other type of pre-diabetes called "impaired glucose tolerant." This form of pre-diabetes is more difficult to diagnose because it requires a longer, 2-hour test known as an oral glucose tolerance test or OGTT (see side panel on next page for more info on this). If your blood sugar is ≥ 140 and < 200 mg/dl at the 2-hour mark while having an OGTT, this is impaired glucose tolerant, also known as pre-diabetes.

	Fasting	After two hours
Normal blood sugar	<100 mg/dl	<140 mg/dl
Impaired Fasting Glucose (IFG)	100-125 mg/dl	
Impaired Glucose Tolerant (IGT)		≥140-199 mg/dl
Diabetes	≥126 mg/dl	≥200 mg/dl

Generally, you should have a few risk factors to justify having an OGTT, whereas the fasting glucose (which diagnoses diabetes) is fairly routine during annual doctor visits after a certain age. Risk factors for developing diabetes include being overweight, having a family history of type 2 diabetes, having the skin condition of acanthosis nigricans, or being of a particular ethnic group (Mexican, Hispanic, Indian, African American, for example). If you exhibit two or more risk factors, your clinician may want to order an OGTT to be proactive before the development of diabetes.

Although this chapter was focused upon the development of diabetes due to obesity, being overweight causes a host of other medical problems such as high blood pressure, high cholesterol, high triglycerides (another type of fat in blood), fatty liver, bone disease, sleep apnea, and hiatal hernia. Existing medical problems, such as asthma, worsen as one gets heavier. Additionally, psychosocial conditions such as poor self esteem, depression, and isolation are also common.

What's An OGTT or Oral Glucose Tolerance Test?

It is a test you take fasting (no food for 10 hours) that requires you to drink a carbohydrate load (sugary drink) that challenges your body to see if it can clear the glucose from the blood to an appropriate level after a certain amount of time (2 hours). In other words, you drink this test so it's called "oral." It tests the sugar tolerance or "glucose tolerance" of your body by seeing if the sugar was cleared or not.

The test obtains a fasting glucose, a one-hour glucose (optional), and a two-hour glucose.

The OGTT is the only test currently available that can diagnose one particular form of pre-diabetes known as Impaired Glucose Tolerant or IGT.

The fasting glucose determines if one has Impaired Fasting Glucose or IFG, which is another form of pre-diabetes. You can have a fasting glucose tested without the full OGTT, however. It is the 2-hour result that clinicians are interested in when they prescribe an OGTT.

PART THREE:

Where You're at and
What You Need to Know
(Assessing and Learning)

CHAPTER 5:

Are You Ready to Make Changes?

Every passing minute is another chance to turn it all around.
~~ From Vanilla Sky.

Why would I designate an entire chapter to whether or not someone is ready to make changes in their lifestyle? Because technically you really *need* to be ready to make changes. Lifestyle modification is extremely difficult. On the other hand, making small modifications in your lifestyle does not require a lot of effort. That is why I feel so strongly about making one or two changes versus ten changes. If you are not ready and you attempt to make ten lifestyle changes and do not succeed, you will probably feel worse than before you started.

Charles F. Wetherall once wrote, "Every diet carries with it the seeds of failure or success. Whether you win or lose is largely a matter of your own will. And where there's a will, there's a way." In other words, if you want something bad enough, you find a way to do it. I do agree that there are people so motivated to lose weight that nothing stops them, I've seen many of them. They are an inspiration to myself and many others.

When I was in the commercial weight loss industry as a young woman beginning my career, the company I worked for called the motivating reason you wanted to lose weight your "hot button." This was the determining factor that caused the client to call the 1-800 phone number and ask for help.

Being the recipient of an insensitive comment was the most common reason that overweight individuals walked through the doorway of the weight loss company. Spouses are typically those who make insensitive comments to each other regarding weight. Many times, the spouse is simply trying to be honest to his or her loved one. I cannot tell you how many times women, in particular, have asked their husbands, "Honey, how do I look in this outfit?" and the poor *#@~ answers very honestly and has no idea of the ramifications of his reply. Another popular reason for deciding to lose weight is not fitting into your pants (the last straw!) or going shopping and leaving discouraged because there are no stylish clothes in your size or you realize you have grown to the next size. I'll never forget that one man who told me he could not fit into the seat at the movie theatre and felt mortified. This man was ready to lose weight. I have heard numerous stories about specific motivating factors for weight loss.

What is truly motivating you? Clearly those who try to lose weight because *they* want to and not because someone else wants them to, do much better. When *you* really want to do it, you are willing to put more effort into it. Many people fail to think about how much effort is involved in changing lifestyle. Although my advice of making small changes does not require a lot of sacrifice or effort, a good practice to determine if you are ready to make any effort to lose weight is to think about the pros and cons of losing weight. A pro might be that you will fit into your favorite pair of jeans again, while a con might be that you have to give up eating ice cream every evening during your favorite TV show. Take a moment to write down some "good things" and "not-so-good or inconvenient things" that will happen while trying to lose weight.

	Good Things	Not-so-good or "inconvenient" Things
Example:	1. I can cross my legs.	1. No more cream and sugar in my coffee.
	2. My diabetes will improve.	2. Need to fit in 30 minutes of exercise each day.
Your answers:	1._____	1._____
	2._____	2._____
	3._____	3._____
	4._____	4._____

This practice gets you thinking about how much work is involved in your new endeavor. Can I really give up the cream and sugar in my coffee? Do I really think that I will exercise 30 minutes every day? What if I work late one night? What if I'm tired? These kinds of questions help you determine if you are truly ready or not.

You will want to balance out the positive factors that may occur as a result of weight loss as well. Think about how your life may improve if you were to lose weight. I often hear patients say that they will be able to cross their legs when sitting down. Will you sleep better in the evening? Will your high blood pressure and/or blood sugar improve? Will you be more alert or confident at work? The list goes on and on...

Your attitude about the effort behind weight loss plays a big role in success. In the example given above about giving up cream and sugar in your coffee, you might resolve that it is not so bad if you switch to 1% milk and an artificial sweetener. This kind of positive attitude goes a long way. Let's face it, weight management is a lifelong commitment and like anything else, your attitude can make it or break it.

I ask all of my patients to think about the pros and cons carefully and then to rate their motivation level on a scale of 1 to 10. Ten is: I want to lose weight now and I'll do whatever it takes. One is: I guess it would be a good idea if I lost weight. Where do you fall on this scale of 1 to 10? Keep track of your motivation level. Does it change? Ask yourself where you are on the scale from time to time.

Date: Motivation Level:

_____   1 2 3 4 5 6 7 8 9 10

_____   1 2 3 4 5 6 7 8 9 10

_____   1 2 3 4 5 6 7 8 9 10

Dr. Kelly Brownell, a psychologist and renowned researcher in the area of weight management from Yale University, developed a questionnaire to use on his patients to determine if they were ready to lose weight. He carried out a study with this questionnaire to determine if readiness mattered. Those that showed readiness to lose weight, indeed, were much more successful at weight loss than those that indicated a lack of readiness to lose weight.

If it is a stressful time in your life, it may make more sense to wait to lose weight. On the contrary, if it is a special time in your life (ready to leave for a cruise, getting married in a few days or weeks, etc.), this may also warrant waiting to shed a few pounds. Significant life issues may interfere with the required effort. My suggestion to you if either of these scenarios describes you is to make one small change and hold off on any major lifestyle changes. If there is more time to start planning for a special event (taking a cruise in six months, getting married in a year, for example), I would also suggest finding one change to make, because one change will make a difference and you have lots of time to see the difference in lifestyle take effect.

In summary, readiness to lose weight is a major factor in weight loss success. Being honest with yourself about willingness to change lifestyle and your attitude are key components to readiness. Shoot for small changes if it is not a good time to make major lifestyle changes.

CHAPTER 6:

The Ins and Outs (calories in and out) of Weight Loss

Losing weight occurs from expending more energy than you consume. The equation, in simplest terms, is:

Energy In (calories) − Energy Out (activity) = Energy Excess (weight gain) or
Energy Deficit (weight loss).

Calories equal energy. Food supplies calories. And calories are necessary to keep your body functioning, including your metabolism. If you cut your calories, you are going to lose weight. This is why many of these fad diets work: overall, they are a restriction of calories. The food prescribed on a fad diet does not perform magic in any way or burn fat simply by consuming it; although that is certainly what most people think. If you went on the banana split diet, you'd lose weight. Two small banana splits each day total fewer calories than what people usually eat from regular meals and snacks.

When you eat excess calories—that is, more calories than your body needs to do its job—you gain weight. Body fat is simply stored calories. This came in handy years ago when we were hunters starving in between outings to catch game. It is hard to starve today in between jaunts to Dunkin Donuts for breakfast and McDonald's for lunch.

Calories have a bad reputation. We instantly think of calories as something bad. How many calories are in that chocolate dessert? Calories, however, are another term for energy. Energy isn't bad, it's good for us. I should say, "It's how you use it that matters." Problems occur when we abuse calories.

To function properly, our bodies require a certain number of calories every day. This number of calories is extremely individualized—it depends on gender, age, activity level, and your own metabolic rate. About 60 to 75 percent of daily caloric needs come from our *resting* metabolic rate which performs functions such as maintaining body temperature, breathing, and heart rate. About 10 percent of daily calorie needs come from eating (great, we burn calories when we eat!), digesting, and absorbing the food we consume. *Basal* energy expenditure is a word used to include both resting energy expenditure and other regular functions such as the eating, digesting, and absorbing of food we just mentioned. The remainder of our caloric needs are due to the *energy* we need for activities such as walking the dog, playing with our kids or grandchildren, gardening, etc.

Formulas exist for dietitians and doctors to help calculate their patient's caloric needs, but these equations are simply a rule of thumb. If you are not a math geek or simply despise math, go directly to #3. These rules of thumb are as follows:

1. Recommended Dietary Allowance (RDA) for energy: 35 calories per kilogram of body weight is the body's weight maintenance requirement. You would then subtract 500 calories per day from this total if you would like to lose weight (500 calories X 7 days per week = 3500 calories = 1 pound of fat per week).

    This is not an accurate method for obese individuals. It tends to overestimate energy needs because it does not account for inactive fat weight. It needs to be adjusted, which gets complicated. To adjust your body weight, you need to know your "healthy" weight, which we discussed in Chapter 1. You can also determine healthy body weight with the BMI chart in Chapter 3. Subtract "healthy" weight from actual weight to determine fat weight. Then multiply fat weight by .25 since fat is less active than muscle. Add this weight to the healthy weight to get your *adjusted body weight*. For example, let's say you are a man that weighs 230 pounds but your healthy weight is 180. 230-180 = 50 pounds excess weight X .25 = 12.50. Add 13 (round up) to 180 to equal 193 pounds. Use this *adjusted body weight* for the equation. 193/2.2 kg per pound = 88 kilograms X 35 calories per kilogram = 3,080 or 3,000 calories. Now (last step) deduct at least 500 calories to produce a caloric deficit. You need approximately 2,400 or 2,500 calories per day. Start here and adjust as needed (if no weight loss after one week, deduct more calories; if too much weight loss, add more calories).

By now, you are most likely appreciating the help of a dietitian. If this was too much information, go directly to #3, don't give up!

2. Basal Energy Expenditure (BEE) equation (Harris-Benedict formula): this is the most formal way to determine energy needs. This is often used in a hospital setting (inpatient where the patient is staying overnight at the hospital) to determine the patient's caloric needs.

BEE (men) = 66 + (13.7 x wt. in kg) + (5 x ht. in cm) – (6.8 x age in yrs)
BEE (women) = 655 + (9.6 x wt. in kg) + (1.7 x ht. in cm) – (4.7 x age in yrs)

After you have calculated BEE, add the activity factor as follows:

Sedentary	Add 20%
Moderate	Add 35%
Active	Add 50%

Terms Used

kg = kilogram
cm = centimeter

BEE = basal energy expenditure
RDA = recommended dietary allowance. See chapter 7 for full description.

Time for an example: Let's say you are a 54-year-old woman, 5' 4" and 200 pounds. First of all, change your wt in pounds to kg by dividing your weight in pounds by 2.2 (200/2.2 = 91 kg). Next change your height in inches to centimeters by multiplying inches by 2.54 (64" X 2.54 = 163 cm).

Here we go: 655 + (9.6 x 91) + (1.7 x 163) – (4.7 x 54) = BEE
        = 655 + 874 + 277 – 254
        = 1806 – 254
        = 1552 calories for BEE

Now add activity factor (.20 for sedentary) = 1552 X .20 = 310 more calories needed for activity = 1552 + 310 = 1,862 Total daily caloric needs

Again, if this woman wants to lose weight, she should deduct at least 500 calories from her total daily caloric needs. This would be 1,362 calories recommended for weight loss.

If you are completely baffled by the above equations, don't despair. See # 3 below.

3. Very crude equation (better known as "The Quick and Dirty Way"): Add a zero to whatever weight you are trying to achieve. This is roughly the number of calories you need to consume daily to achieve this weight over time. For example, if you would like to weigh 180 pounds, 1800 calories per day is a good start to determine your caloric needs. If you lose too much weight (more than a few pounds per week to start), you need to add more calories. Likewise, if you do not lose weight, create an additional caloric deficit by taking in less calories (say, 1600 calories per day).

    I wish I could take credit for this much simpler approach, but the truth is, Dr. Rosa Hendler, Professor of Endocrinology at Yale University School of Medicine, taught me this. I'll never forget the day she showed me this short cut. As a budding dietitian, I looked up at her in amazement (actually down, because she's shorter, but much smarter than I), surprised that no one at Saint Joseph College, where I attended college, or at Saint Francis Hospital, where I did my dietetics internship, ever showed me this.

    It is generally accepted that women should not consume less than 1,200 calories while dieting and men should not consume less than 1,500 calories while dieting. My recommendations, however, are always higher than this (before you get too excited, they are not a heck of a lot higher). The best way to determine how many calories you need to take in to lose weight is the most time consuming way (# 4 below). You may need a dietitian to help you with this accurate technique.

4. Usual calorie intake with calorie deficit:

    Write down a typical day's worth of food consumption or, more ideally, have a dietitian do a diet recall or typical daily intake with you. It is best if the dietitian asks you about the foods you eat because he/she will know specific questions to ask to gain the most knowledge about the type of food and the calories involved. For example, what kind of milk was it—skim, 1%, 2% or whole? How much milk did you drink—one or two glasses? Were they 8-ounce or 10-ounce cups? How was the chicken prepared—baked or fried? With skin or without the skin? Dietitians are trained to get the most information about the food you have consumed and to provide the most accurate caloric intakes. He or she may also ask you to describe both a typical weekday and weekend intake since these two types of days tend to be very different. An average of the two types of days may be calculated to determine the average daily intake.

There are several books and phone apps on the market that list foods with their respective calories. My favorite book for looking up nutrient composition and calories is *Bowe's and Church's Food Values of Portions Commonly Used* (Pennington J.A. and Spungen J, 2010). There are many pocket size books that simply list calories, however some also include grams of carbohydrate or fat since some people count carbs or fat, but not calories. It is a huge undertaking to look up each food and beverage that you consume for three days (two week days and one weekend day) to get an estimate of your usual daily caloric intake (add the total of three days and then divide by three to get your average daily intake). The available apps or the help of a dietitian can be extremely time saving to you. What may take you hours and hours adding up, the dietitian can add up in his or her head in minutes or the app can total in seconds (we are being replaced—not really!). I recommend, however, that you use either a book or app with calorie values to look up foods in general to help you become more aware of the caloric values of foods.

Once you know how many calories you typically consume in one day, you should subtract about 500 calories (or a bit more if your calorie intake is quite high) per day from this usual daily total.

When we eat fewer calories than our bodies require, the stored fat gets paid a visit and viola, we lose fat (weight)! To lose one pound of fat, we have to reduce our caloric consumption by 3,500 calories. In case you skipped over to this chapter before reading chapter one, go back and read my examples of how easy it is to overeat on 3,500 calories! There I give examples of small daily behaviors that add up (I also give calorie-saving examples in Chapter 10) Here I will tell you that one typical fast food meal supplies over 1700 calories (that's one meal). Hello pounds! One fettucine alfredo meal with dessert supplies about 2,000 calories. I think I've said enough. I don't have to tell you that it is extremely easy in this day and age to take in too many calories.

I like to think of the weight loss equation as this: Food in − Exercise out = Weight gain/loss. Up to this point we've talked about the calories consumed. The good news is that you do burn calories every day. When you do something structured for a specific amount of time, you can rely on X number of calories to be burned. Maybe you can go to the gym for 40 minutes every day, maybe you can play tennis every Saturday. This is structured exercise. Also, I am a fan of "here and there" exercise. We always have time for this kind of exercise. Here and There exercise is volunteering to go into the convenience store versus waiting in the car, taking the stairs versus the elevator at work, getting up to change the channel versus using the remote, or hanging your laundry on a clothes line versus throwing them in the dryer (we'll get into more examples in Chapter 11). Anyway, all of these movements—big or small, structured or non-structured—add up to caloric use. What we are striving for in weight loss is a caloric deficit (you want to be in the red) at the end of the day.

That's it, there is no magic; it's called caloric deficit. Does it matter what you eat? Absolutely. The banana split diet doesn't have all the nutrients we need on a daily basis. Do you remember the food groups you learned in elementary school? There is a reason for these food groups. Any time a crash or fad diet promises wonderful things, always ask yourself if all of the food groups are present in it. If it is missing a food group, it is missing at least one important nutrient. There is a reason why dietitians say to eat a variety of foods. The challenge at weight loss is trying to obtain all the nutrition you need for the fewest calories—this means you will need to eat a variety of foods.

CHAPTER 7:

Nutrition 101 and Donuts 540

Get your facts first, then you can distort them as you please.
~~Mark Twain

You may be a novice at nutrition, but a graduate student at eating donuts. Been there, done that! Remind me to tell you about me and donuts; we go way back! My philosophy as a dietitian does not require that you never eat a sweet again (how awful!). I am not your typical dietitian by any means. I do think there is room in everyone's diet for fun food. Do you remember I said earlier that it's all in the way you use it? This certainly applies to sweets or other "junk" foods.

Before I keep referring to junk food, let's take a look at some basic nutrition facts so that the term junk food can be appreciated. Take a look at the words for nutrients I have listed. Here you will find a simple explanation for each one. Basically, there are macronutrients (big nutrients) and micronutrients (little nutrients). Macronutrients have energy or calories, micronutrients do not. Micronutrients are vitamins and elements that help the macronutrients function efficiently or work with other micronutrients to perform vital body functions. Carbohydrate, protein, and fat are macronutrients. Carbohydrate and protein are each 4 calories per gram, while fat is 9 calories per gram (you can easily see why high-fat foods are higher in calories than lower fat foods).

Macronutrients or "Big" Nutrients with Calories

Carbohydrate – The principal role of carbohydrate is to provide energy for the body and heat to maintain body temperature. The central nervous system (brain) and lens of the eye can only use glucose (building blocks for carbohydrate) for energy, but other tissues can also use fat.

Protein – The primary role of protein is to build and repair body tissues. A secondary role is to provide energy. Amino acids are the building blocks for proteins.

Fat – This macronutrient is a concentrated source of energy, furnishing 9 calories per gram in comparison to 4 calories per gram in the other two macronutrients. Important fat-soluble vitamins found in foods could not be transported throughout the intestinal tract and absorbed if fat was not consumed.

Carbohydrates are generally foods such as fruit, milk, vegetables, sugar, and grains and starches such as pasta, bread, and rice. Proteins are primarily fish, chicken, beef, cheese, and legumes. Fats probably do not need very much explaining. They are foods such as butter, margarine, oil, salad dressing, mayonnaise, cream cheese, olives, and visible fat on meat. This is a very abbreviated list because if you have every dieted before, you probably know this basic information.

You may also know that many foods do not fall neatly into one macronutrient category, but are a mixture of two or three. For example, beans are high in both carbohydrate and a protein. Nuts are high in protein and fat, but also have some carbohydrate in them. The composition of macronutrients in our daily diets is suggested to be as follows: 55 percent of our calories from carbohydrate, 15 percent from protein, and 30 percent or less from fat.

Micronutrients or "Little" Nutrients with no calories, but special jobs

This is not a full list, but I want to give you an idea of some micronutrients and their role in the body:

Vitamin A – fat-soluble vitamin that helps keep our cell membranes and nerve cells healthy. It aids hormones such as cortisol and thyroxin, assists in immune reactions, and helps manufacture red blood cells.

Vitamin B – water-soluble vitamins that maintain the integrity of the central nervous system. There are several B vitamins: B_1 or Thiamin; B_2 or riboflavin; B_3 or niacin; B_6 or pyridoxine; and B_{12}. B_2 and B_6 are also involved in protein metabolism, while B_{12} is essential for the normal function of all body cells and red blood cell maturation.

Vitamin C – water-soluble vitamin that maintains the integrity of capillaries, promotes healing of wounds and fractures, aids with tooth and bone formation, and increases iron absorption.

Vitamin D – fat-soluble vitamin that helps mineralize bones and teeth and regulates blood calcium levels. This vitamin is intricately related to calcium and phosphorus (each being required for utilization of the other).

Vitamin E – fat-soluble vitamin that acts as an antioxidant, protecting the integrity of normal cell membranes. It also protects Vitamin A and assists in the prevention of red blood cell breakdown.

Vitamin K – fat- and water-soluble vitamin that is necessary in the blood-clotting process.

Calcium – an element responsible for bone and tooth formation, and appropriate calcium balance in the body, including the blood. Calcium is stored in the bone but is called upon when the blood needs it for special functions such as nerve impulses, muscle contraction and relaxation, blood clotting, structure and function of cell membranes, and absorption of vitamin B_{12}.

Phosphorus – an element that works closely with calcium. A sufficient phosphorus intake is necessary to avoid a loss of calcium as it helps absorb calcium. There is a reciprocal relationship between these two minerals: If calcium levels are low, phosphorus increases in the blood to increase calcium's absorption. However, if blood calcium levels become too high, phosphorus levels go down so less calcium is absorbed (too much calcium can create a stone formation).

Iron – an element needed by the bone marrow to form hemoglobin for red blood cells. This mineral also transports oxygen from the lungs to the tissues and brings forth many oxidative reactions within cells, including a final step needed for energy metabolism.

Folic Acid – a water-soluble vitamin that is important during pregnancy for proper DNA formulation. Another primary role is the formation of heme, the iron part of hemoglobin in the red blood cell. Folic acid needs vitamin C. In fact, it is folacin before it becomes folic acid and without vitamin C, it cannot convert to its biologically active form called folic acid. This is another example of how these micronutrients need each other.

Potassium – an element that works in conjunction with sodium to maintain the balance of fluids in our body. You may have heard potassium referred to as an electrolyte.

Magnesium – an element important in controlling normal heart function. Besides calcium and phosphorus, bones contain most of the body's magnesium. Magnesium has many functions, including an enzyme action vital to the production of energy, calcium and phosphorus metabolism in bone, and integrity of heart muscles and other muscles and nerves.

Nutrient-dense and Junk Foods

Junk foods can be defined as empty-calorie foods. What does empty-calorie mean? It 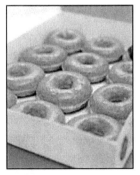 means that you get a lot of calories for very little or no nutritional value. A donut is an excellent example. Let's take a yummy cream donut. This treat has approximately 450 calories and gives us only fat and carbohydrate (sugar), no vitamins, no minerals, no protein.

The opposite of a junk food is a nutrient-dense food. An apple is an excellent example of this. A medium apple is approximately 100 calories. For 100 calories, you get Vitamin A, potassium, fiber, and a little bit of Vitamin C as well. An apple is all carbohydrate, no fat or protein. An 8-ounce glass of skim milk has 90 calories. For 90 calories, you get calcium, riboflavin, Vitamin D, protein and carbohydrate. Now that's a deal!

Time for another definition: Low-fat and High-fat foods. As you can see, a low-fat food derives less than 30% of its total calories from fat, while a high-fat food derives greater than 30% of its total calories from fat. Incidentally, if a food is high-fat, particularly if it is a snack food, it is also considered a junk food. Let's figure out an example. Can you think of another junk food (duh!)? Let's take sour cream and onion potato chips. The serving size is one ounce, but let's be serious, who eats an ounce of potato chips. Let's be a bit more realistic by estimating our serving as two ounces (keep it to yourself if you generally eat ½ a bag!). Two ounces of chips have 300 calories, 29 grams of carb, and 20 grams of fat. Some manufacturers will indicate that there is vitamin C (due to the potatoes), but the vitamin C you get—10 to 20% daily value (check definitions for this)—is not worth all of the fat. This is clearly a high-fat food since there are 20 grams of fat and 300 total calories (20 grams of fat X 9 calories per gram = 180 calories derived from fat; 180 ÷ 300 total calories = 60% calories from fat). This is also a junk food because the nutrients you get (Vitamin C) are not worth the high amount of fat.

Similar to the potato chip example, there are lots of foods that may have one good nutrient in them, but they are still terribly high in fat or sugar. What about a chocolate bar? A typical 1 ½ ounce chocolate bar has about 230 calories and gives us fat and carbohydrate. Wait a minute…I should mention that there is a tad of calcium, iron, and magnesium in chocolate (I look for every excuse to eat it). In all honesty, there's not enough of these minerals to qualify this baby as a nutrient-dense food, but you can't blame a girl for trying! There are 13 grams or more of fat in this 1 ½ ounce chocolate bar. Now let's go back to the total calories of 230. Multiple the number of fat grams by 9 to give us fat calories and we get 117 calories from fat. Now divide the fat calories by the total calories and we get 51% calories from fat. It's a darn shame.

On the flip side, there are low-fat foods available to us. Fruits and vegetables fit this description nicely. We already figured out above that an apple is pure carbohydrate with lots of wonderful micronutrients. No fat to be found. Broccoli has zero fat and is primarily all carb (a little bit of protein) with lots of vitamin A, Vitamin C, folic acid, potassium, fiber, and some calcium as well. What a wonderful choice! A low-fat food doesn't have to be a

---

Terms Used

Empty-calorie food = food with little or no nutritional value

Nutrient-dense food = food rich in nutritional value

High fat foods =
> 30% of the food's calorie is from fat
Low fat foods =
< 30% of the food's calorie is from fat

Recommended Daily Allowance (also called Recommended Dietary Allowance) = how much you need of a nutrient on average every day if you are a healthy individual.

Adequate Intake = when there is not enough scientific evidence to determine a RDA, an AI is developed

Percent Daily Value = the % of a particular nutrient obtained from a food (based on a total daily calorie need of 2,000 calories per day)

fruit or vegetable, however. Let's look at two types of crackers:

Soda-type cracker (better known as a Saltine) vs. Butter-type cracker (i.e., Ritz):

	Soda cracker	butter cracker
Serving size	4	4
Fat (grams)	1	4
Carbohydrate (grams)	9	9
Protein (grams)	1	1
Total calories	50	75
% calories from fat	18%	48%
(fat cals/total cals)		

Clearly the soda cracker is a low-fat choice, while the butter-type is a high-fat choice. There are low-fat Ritz crackers on the market today, but there is no reason for the food manufacturers of Saltines to make a low-fat version since it already is.

Since I am a firm believer in short cuts to complex methods, there is an easier method than above: For every 100 calories, a food should have 3 grams or less to be considered low-fat. If it has more than 3 grams of fat per 100 calories, it is considered high-fat. Why didn't I tell you this earlier? Like everything else, it helps you understand the concept when you learn the complete method first.

One more complicating concept to grasp: A food can be low-fat and still be a junk food. And a food can be high-fat, but be nutrient-dense. The later is less common. Let's take a look at a low-fat, junk food such as licorice. Licorice is low-fat, but empty calories (all sugar and no nutrients). Do kids eat licorice today? I have a feeling I am dating myself. Maybe I should refer to more popular candy such as Gummy Bears, Swedish Fish, Sour Patch Kids, or Air Heads instead (I have a 6-year-old, I swear!). All of these sugar-based candies are the same: junk food. It is common for some to think that these are acceptable choices since they are fat-free. I suppose if you had to watch your total fat very carefully and you had to choose between a candy that is high in fat (chocolate bar) versus a candy that is low in fat but very high in sugar, the sugar-based candy might be slightly better.

An example of a nutrient-dense food that is high in fat would be peanut butter. This food is rich in protein, vitamin E, niacin, and also provides iron, but is very high in fat. If you use it sparingly, it's a fine food. Peanut butter on celery is a healthy snack for adults or kids. A peanut butter sandwich is still a superior choice for lunch over fast food or hot lunch.

I would like to explain two important terms: Recommended Dietary Allowances (RDAs) and Adequate Intakes (AIs). A Recommended Dietary Allowance or RDA is a recommended intake of a specific nutrient to provide for individual variations among most healthy people in the United States. For example, a 40-year-old woman needs 1,000 mg of calcium each day. This is her RDA for calcium. These values change based upon gender and age.

When a RDA is recommended, enough research has been done on the nutrient to recommend a specific amount. On the other hand, an Adequate Intake or AI may be assigned to a nutrient, but scientific evidence is still lacking. There is continuous research being done to find out what appropriate nutrient requirements are for various age groups. Even the RDA can change if enough current studies support more or less of a vitamin or element. In fact, before 1998 we simply had RDAs, but responding to the vast knowledge we have today regarding the roles of nutrients in health, the Food and Nutrition Board of the Institute of Medicine has updated these RDAs, included the term AI, and now refers to the two terms as Dietary References Intakes or DRIs.

For your convenience, I have included the DRIs for vitamins and elements in Appendices A.1. and A.2., respectively. There are a series of DRIs that can be found at www.nap.edu. However, the specifics of these reports are beyond the scope of this book.

Lastly, I would like to explain the term Percent Daily Value. It is a bit more "user-friendly" than RDA or AI. This term was established for label reading. It is convenient to compare foods' nutrient density by comparing their percent daily value. It also helps determine if a food is a "junk food." If there are all zeroes next to the nutrients listed, the food is most likely an empty calorie food.

Listed below are both nutrient-dense and empty-calorie snack foods. Notice that the nutrient-dense snack choices have values beside the term "percent daily value" found on the food label. Empty-calorie snack choices are low on nutrients and often high in sugar and/or fat. To determine if something is high in sugar, the total carbohydrates will equal or be close to the amount of sugar listed on the label. An additional method to determine if a food is high in sugar is to look at the first three ingredients listed on the package, bottle, or carton. Is sugar or some other form of sugar (sucrose, dextrose, glucose, fructose, high fructose corn syrup) at the beginning of the list of ingredients? If it is, the food is most likely a poor nutritional choice. You may want to check other brand names, however, as ingredients can vary between food companies for a similar type of food. Yogurt is a good example of ingredient differences between companies.

Here are some nutrient-dense snack choices:

Mozzarella Cheese Sticks
Ingredients: pasteurized part skim milk, cheese cultures, salt, enzymes.

Serving Size:	stick
Calories	90
Calories from fat	50
Total fat	6 g
Total Carbohydrate	1 g
Dietary fiber	0 g
Sugars	0 g
Protein	8 g
Vitamin A	2%
Calcium	20%
Vitamin C	0%
Iron	0%

Stonyfield Yogurt (fat-free), vanilla
Ingredients: cultured pasteurized organic non-fat milk, naturally milled organic sugar, organic natural vanilla flavor, pectin, vitamin D3, six live active cultures.

Serving Size:	6 oz.
Calories	130
Calories from fat	0
Total fat	0 g
Total Carbohydrate	25 g

Dietary fiber	0 g
Sugars	24 g
Protein	7 g
Vitamin A	0%
Calcium	30%
Vitamin C	0%
Vitamin D	20%
Iron	0%

Here are some empty-calorie snack choices:

Oreo Cookies
Ingredients: sugar, enriched flour, riboflavin (B2), folic acid, high oleic canola oil and/or palm oil and/or canola oil, and/or soybean oil, cocoa (processed with alkali), high fructose corn syrup, cornstarch, leavening (baking soda and/or calcium phosphate), salt, soy lecithin (emulsifier), vanillin – an artificial flavor, chocolate.

Serving Size:	3 cookies
Calories	160
Calories from fat	65
Total fat	7.0 g
Total Carbohydrate	25.0 g
Dietary fiber	1.0 g
Sugars	14.0 g
Protein	1 g
Vitamin A	0%
Calcium	2%
Vitamin C	0%
Iron	10%

Cheese Doodles
Ingredients: corn meal, vegetable oil, whey, salt, corn starch, calcium carbonate, buttermilk, cheddar cheese, monosodium glutamate, artificial color, milk, calcium, sodium caseinate, butter oil, yellow 6 lake, yellow 5 lake, lactic acid, natural flavors.

Serving Size:	1 oz.
Calories	160
Calories from fat	90
Total fat	10 g
Total Carbohydrate	13 g
Dietary fiber	0 g
Sugars	<1 g
Protein	2 g
Vitamin A	0%
Calcium	0%
Vitamin C	0%
Iron	2%

Although the cheese stick is high in fat (more than 50% of the calories come from fat, 50 calories from fat ÷ 90 total calories = 55%), it offers protein and calcium. This is a healthy choice as long as you don't abuse these foods (i.e., you don't eat three or four in one sitting). This food is very much like peanut butter—high in fat but rich in other important nutrients—which we've already discussed.

The yogurt is a wonderful choice. A portion of one's calcium requirement can be obtained for as little as 140 calories. Additionally the choice is low in fat (9% calories from fat) and has 7 grams of protein (1/3 of the protein in a 3-ounce burger).

Oreo cookies, on the other hand, are not a good choice. With one gram of protein and a whopping 7 grams of fat, this food is not a nutritional bargain. The only positive statement is that it offers 10% iron and, overall, this is not a good way to obtain iron (meat, legumes, and green vegetables are a more nutritional bargain for iron).

Cheese Doodles are even worse than Oreos because they are higher in fat and offer less iron (2% dietary allowance) for the same calories per serving. Other than being low in sugar, I cannot find a good thing to say about the food.

By the way, junk foods are usually high in fat or sugar. Why? Because (a) these things make the food taste good and (b) these things preserve the food. Sometimes foods are also high in salt for the same reasons. That's why a low-fat food is typically higher in sugar than its original version, and there is usually a higher salt content as well.

Too Much (Junk Food), Too Often!

OK, enough of Nutrition 101. We will discuss loads of better food choices in Chapter 10, "1 Thing" Ideas: Making Better Food Choices. Let's talk about Donuts 540. I think there is room in our diet for occasional junk food. My belief about high-sugar or high-fat foods is that we can enjoy these products in moderation. The cookies, snacks, and sugar candies discussed earlier can be enjoyed by children (and parents) once in a while. Life is too short to always mind your Ps and Qs. How many people could actually say that they don't enjoy going to the ice cream parlor?...the donut shop (now you're talking my language)?..., or the pizza parlor? We all deserve to have a little fun and should. It's when we abuse junk food that we get into trouble.

When I was a senior in high school, my favorite thing to do after school was to go to the donut shop with a particular friend. I am embarrassed to say how many donuts we would eat in one sitting and I am further embarrassed to tell you how often we visited this shop. If you think I don't know what it is to be overweight and what it is to feel completely out of control around food, you don't know enough about me.

I started gaining weight rapidly in my senior year of high school. My parents were going through a divorce and I found comfort in overeating. The foods I chose to overeat were not foods that were healthy (why don't we ever turn to celery sticks when we are having a bad day?). However, the comfort I experienced was only temporary, as you may already know from your own experience. This fleeting moment of solace was soon followed by guilt and sadness. Many times I would also feel physically uncomfortable because I didn't overeat a little, I ate until I felt the familiar feeling in my stomach that implied I couldn't eat another thing. My stomach felt expanded to its capacity, but I had become accustomed to the feeling.

To give you an idea of how quickly one can gain weight from eating junk food, let's say that I ate four donuts per day (I ate more than this, however). Let's use a glazed donut of 250 calories for the sake of simplicity. This is an extra 1,000 *per day*! In just one week, I would gain 2 pounds! Remember, an extra 3500 calories equates to a pound of fat. No wonder I gained weight so rapidly.

Hopefully you have not experienced overeating to this degree. Some overeating is completely normal and you should forgive yourself and move on. The trick is to learn the triggers that lead you to the overeating. We will cover this in Chapters 12 (Becoming More Aware) and 13 (Taming of the Shrew). Had I understood how to identify triggers and deal with them, I certainly would not have overeaten as much as I did.

CHAPTER 8:

Get Up Off the Sofa!

If it weren't for the fact that the TV set and the refrigerator are far apart,
some of us wouldn't get any exercise at all.
~~Joey Adams

What would you say if I told you that from a health perspective, exercise is just as important as good nutrition and sleep? That's right, sleep! Most people reply to me, "Boy, I've got a lot of exercising to catch up on."

Think of these three components—exercise, good nutrition, and sleep—as a triangle to weight management. One cannot work without the other. If you don't get enough sleep, you will most likely make poor food choices and certainly not have the energy to exercise. If you don't make good food choices, you will most likely not feel like exercising. When we don't get enough exercise, we often find it hard to go to sleep because the body is not physically tired enough. We will revisit this triangle concept in the next chapter.

As we learned in Chapter 7, exercise contributes to the output side of the energy balance equation:

Energy In (calories) – Energy Out (activity) = Energy Excess (weight gain) or
Energy Deficit (weight loss)

In addition to helping one lose weight, exercise has many other benefits:

- Fights depression
- Helps change fat to muscle
- Makes our heart stronger
- Improves the "good" cholesterol
- Slows down the aging process

Exercise releases chemicals known as endorphins which are natural tranquilizers. When we engage in activity, these chemicals are released into the blood stream. If your weight problem has you feeling sad, the best thing you can do is become active.

As you can imagine, the ratio of fat to muscle changes with exercise. Fat gets used up with sustained exercise (see below). An important muscle in the body is our heart. The heart becomes more efficient at pumping oxygen and blood when we exercise regularly. It gets even better: the good cholesterol or high-density lipoproteins (HDL) improves with exercise. HDL nourishes the blood. Also, fat levels in the blood known as triglycerides decrease with exercise. HDL and triglycerides are opposites. Generally speaking, when one goes up, the other goes down and vice versa. We want the HDL to go up and the triglycerides to go down.

Exercise slows down the aging process. It increases oxygen consumption, bringing more blood flow to the body. It slows down the natural decline in daily energy expenditure as we get older. In addition to physical changes in the body, exercise has shown the ability to preserve cognitive functioning as one ages. In general, quality of life can be better for the middle-aged or older adult when exercise is part of their routine.

Unlike nutrients, there is no RDA (Recommended Dietary Allowance) for how much exercise a typical person should get per day. In general, research suggests that 60 to 90 minutes per day is needed for weight loss and 60 minutes per day for weight maintenance. Sticking to the essence of this book (simplicity), you should understand that if you are trying to lose weight, you will need to get more activity than you are currently experiencing. If you do nothing right now, adding 15 minutes of activity to your daily routine would be helpful. Don't get hung up on the amount of time you exercise for now. Just try to do more than you normally do.

Incidentally, a study published in 2008 in the British Journal of Sports Medicine showed that regular aerobic exercise can slow down the aging process (by up to 12 years!). The study doctor, Dr. Tepper, had studied the effects of only 30 minutes of daily, brisk walking or the equivalent.

There are two forms of exercise: Planned activity and what I call "here and there" exercise. When I go out for a hike, this is a planned activity for me (it also happens to be an enjoyable leisurely activity for me, but we'll talk about the importance of this in a minute). When I park my car in the parking lot at work and walk a bit before I actually sit at my desk, this is "here and there" activity. The trick is to get a lot of "here and there" exercise while finding a structured activity that you enjoy (or can at least tolerate!). For the record, I use the words exercise and activity interchangeably, but one might argue that the word *activity* sounds less painful than the word *exercise*. I hope I don't confuse you, but making this distinction would go against my grain. You can refer to the planned stuff as planned exercise if you wish and the "here and there" stuff as "here and there" activity if it makes more sense to you. My goal is that you use these two words interchangeably as well some day.

Let's talk about "here and there" activity first (baby steps, my dear friend!). Think about your typical day. Do you walk to your car? Take the stairs? Go grocery shopping? Walk outside to get the mail from the mailbox? Walk inside the coffee shop instead of driving through the drive-through window? These are all little bits of exercise that add up by the end of the day. In a minute we will add up Pamela's "here and there" exercise and come up with a total of calories burned in one day.

Here is a list of chores that fall into the "here and there" activities category, but if done for a long time (in other words, you had to plan to do it), the activities could definitely be considered planned activities. Notice the calories burned per hour. However, I will always include the calories burned per 10 minutes because, in case I haven't made it clear, I believe a little is better than nothing:

"Here and There" Activities

	Calories burned/hour	Calories burned/10 min
Cleaning house (general)	180	30
Cleaning (heavy; Washing windows, car)	204	34
Child care (bath, grooming)	204	34
Child care (playing)	340	57
Chopping wood	408	68
Gardening (general)	272	45
Gardening (weeding)	306	51
Laundry	136	23
Mopping	238	40
Mowing lawn (walk, hand-power)	408	68
Mowing lawn (power mower)	306	51
Raking	292	49
Shoveling snow	408	68
Operating snow blower	306	51
Shopping (slow walk)	156	26
Putting away groceries	165	28
Vacuuming	238	40
Walking the dog	230	38
Washing dishes	156	26
My favorite: Having a manicure!	68	11

Now let's talk about planned exercise. The types of exercise that fall into this category might be the following. Again, I have included the calories burned per hour or per 10 minutes:

Planned or Structured Activities

	Calories burned/hour	Calories burned/10 min
Taking a walk	239	40
Walking briskly (treadmill or pavement)	273	46
Taking a hike (climbing upward)	540	90
Riding your bike (leisurely)	273	46
Jogging	477	80
Rollerblading	477	80
Ice Skating	477	80
Dancing (low impact)	341	57
Dancing (general)	409	68
Skiing	477	80
Basketball (non-game)	409	68
Basketball (game)	545	91
Baseball or softball	341	57
Soccer	477	80
Swimming (leisure)	409	68
Swimming (moderate)	545	91
Horseback riding	273	46
Golfing	307	51
Miniature golf	205	34

Some activities might be a mix of the two. For example, is mowing the lawn a planned or "here and there" activity? Based upon the exertion you generally use when you push a lawn mower and the amount of time it takes to mow the lawn, I would put it in the planned category unless you have a rider (we'll have to talk because a rider doesn't even belong in the "here and there" category). Shoveling the snow is definitely a planned activity because it actually requires even more effort than mowing the lawn. Chores generally fall into the "here and there" classification, but I wanted to mention a few of these that were a bit much (I'm not heartless!).

Usually, planned activities involve more exertion than "here and there" activities and burn more calories. It is important to note that all activities that are aerobic (require oxygen) are heart healthy and lead to weight loss. An activity that is non-aerobic is weight lifting, although it does strengthen and bulk muscles. Repeating weight lifting, however, using resistance such as nautilus can be aerobic if it requires more than a quick bit of energy (i.e., if it lasts longer than 90 seconds). Planned activities are generally longer than "here and there" activities, which is another way of differentiating the two.

Sally worked on her computer all day until her friend got home from work and they met to go rollerblading. One hour of rollerblading burned 477 calories. She returned home after rollerblading and watched her favorite sitcom. Pamela, on the other hand, had a busy day which consisted of no planned exercise at all, but the following "here and there" activities:

7:00 – 8:00 AM	Folded 1 load of laundry
	Made lunch for family
	Straightened up the kitchen
	Vacuumed the 1st floor of the house
8:00 – 8:15 AM	Ran after and dressed toddler
8:30 AM	Walked 3 minutes from parking garage to office
11:30 AM	Took the stairs 4 flights up and 4 down to deliver document at work
1:00 PM	Walked to meet a friend for a quick lunch at nearby park (5-minute walk)
4:00 PM	Parked car a bit further in grocery store lot and shopped for a total of 25 minutes (dinner ingredients, etc.)
4:30 PM	Picked up child at daycare (in and out of car, etc.) (husband dropped child off in AM, what a guy!!)
4:45 PM	Picked up dry cleaning (in and out of car, etc.)
5:00 PM	Put groceries away and kept up with toddler while trying to cook dinner

7:00 PM	Cleaned dinner dishes and straightened kitchen again
7:45 PM	Folded another load of laundry while watching TV and playing with toddler
8:15 PM	Bathed and put toddler to bed
8:45 PM	Relaxed!!

Do you think Sally or Pamela burned more calories by 9:00 PM? Theoretically, total calories burned were close for both women (800 to 900 calories), which proves that small bursts of exercise can equal longer durations. The advantage that Sally has over Pam is that she had more of a cardiovascular workout and burned more fat with the sustained activity.

If doing sustained activity (not "here and there"), check your heart rate to be sure you are in the "training mode." See "Estimating Maximum Heart Rate" section below to see what your maximum heart rate should be. If you are working over this maximum rate, you will not be getting the cardiovascular benefits of staying within the range for your age.

Estimating Maximum Heart Rate

You can estimate your maximum heart rate by subtracting your age from 220. For example, if you are 40 years old, your maximum heart rate equals 180.

Now take 70% of this number to find the level for a cardiovascular training effort. For example 180 X .70 = 126 beats per minute. This is the number of beats you need to try to feel (I'll explain how below) in one minute. Watching the clock for 15 seconds is a much quicker method, however, than counting for a full minute. This 40-year-old should obtain approximately 31 or 32 beats in 15 seconds to obtain an efficient training rate.

How to Take Your Pulse (beats per minute):

1. Select either wrist or the right side of your neck.
2. If wrist: Wrap fingers of other hand around back of wrist. Press

the index and middle fingers on the upturned wrist until you feel the regular pulsing of the blood through the vessel. If right side of neck: Using your index and middle finger, find the area of your neck that is between under your chin and under your ears. Feel around for a regular pulsing of the blood through the vessel.

3. Count the number of beats (pulses) in exactly 15 seconds. If someone else is not counting for you, look at the second hand of a clock.
4. Multiply the number by 4 to calculate your beats per minute.

If the above-mentioned 40-year-old counted 118 beats per minute, he could probably work a little harder provided he has not just started his workout regimen. If the 40-year-old counted 135, he should not exert himself as much.

Do this pulse check when you are resting to see the difference. The average resting pulse rate for adults is approximately 70 beats per minute (divided by 4 for a 15-second count is about 17 or 18).

Try to breathe as normally as possible while working out (yeah, right!). This is a goal to strive for. Regular breathing ensures the best oxygen consumption and, therefore, the best cardiovascular workout. This will come with regular exercise. The fancy word for better heart health is "cardiovascular conditioning" which is characterized by many benefits including increased breathing efficiency, improved circulation, increased blood volume and oxygen delivery, increased heart strength, and reduced blood pressure.

If you recall, we talked about glycogen (Chapter 2) and fatty acids (Chapter 4) earlier. Glycogen is stored glucose which is used for immediate energy needs when there is not enough glucose in the blood. Fatty acids are byproducts of fat breakdown. Fat is used when we exercise for a while and run out of glycogen stores. Our fat stores play a vital role in their ability to give us prolonged energy. After the body uses glycogen, the muscles call on the fatty acids in the blood (yes, the same ones that get in the way of the insulin doing its job correctly). Once the fatty acids in the blood are all used up, fat breakdown begins to occur (I thought that would get your attention!).

Without getting too technical here, I'd also like to note that a hormone epinephrine is released. Epinephrine signals the fat cells to break apart their stored fat (triglycerides) and let lots of fatty acids into the blood. So fat gets used up two ways when you are active: the muscle takes what is in the blood stream but also epinephrine comes to the rescue and tells the fat cells to start breaking down. Aerobic type of exercise allows the best fat consumption as oxygen is used to burn the fat.

Repeated or regular aerobic workouts (even just 20 minutes three or four times per week) stimulate the muscle cells to make tiny little organs (organelles) called mitochondria. If you thought epinephrine was a good guy, you'll be very happy to meet mitochondria, whose job is to get along very well with enzymes that burn fat in the muscle cells. People often ask, "What is more important, the intensity of the workout or the duration?" If you are trying to lose weight, the duration is very important. Persistent, low-intensity exercise—such as fast walking or bicycling—is an excellent way to maximize the use of fat. In general, the longer the duration of activity, the more fat used up for energy consumption.

If exercise helps you to relieve stress, you may choose to exercise later in the day when your stress level is high versus first thing in the morning. Exercising too late, however, may interfere with your sleep as you may get an adrenaline surge, which could keep you up at night. As stated earlier, epinephrine (or adrenaline) is a hormone released in the body during exercise.

The perfect time for me to exercise is about 4:00 or 5:00 p.m., after I have worked all day and built a bit of stress up. I find that the workout really alleviates the stress. The time is also good for me because I haven't eaten dinner yet. There is nothing worse than eating and then exercising shortly after. Everyone is different, however. Many people like to start their day with exercise because it puts them in the right frame of mind. Others prefer working out early in the morning so that it is "over with."

Moral of the story in this chapter: Structured exercise that is aerobic in nature of a 20-minute or longer duration is best for weight loss. "Here and there" exercise is better than "no exercise anywhere" and in some cases more realistic. If you don't move, you won't lose weight. Once you lose weight, you still have to move to keep the weight off! It's well worth it! You will feel better, do your body good (improve cholesterol, fitness level), and change your metabolism by converting fat to muscle. Did I mention that you'll look better, too?

Chapter 11 offers ideas about how exercise can burn calories and how much weight can be lost by adding structured or "here and there" activity to your daily routine.

CHAPTER 9:

Maybe You Should Be Counting Sheep, Not Calories!

I love sleep. My life has a tendency to fall apart when I'm awake, you know?
--Ernest Hemingway

Exercise, eating well, and sleep have a reciprocal relationship. Think of these three things as the angles of a triangle. They rely on each other.

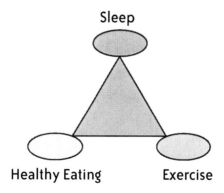

If you don't sleep well, you won't feel like exercising the next day. Most likely, you won't care about eating healthy the next day either. Likewise, if you don't eat healthy, you may not want to exercise (black and white mentality of "oh, I blew it anyway.") Also, when we overeat, we have a hard time sleeping. The feeling of fullness or indigestion may be uncomfortable. Caffeine and high-sodium foods can also create havoc when we lay our heads down on the pillow.

The "one thing" for you, if you do not get enough sleep, may be to go to bed early in the evening. Yes, that's it: go to bed early. If you continually go to bed late and wake up early during the week, only to make up an hour or two on the weekends, you are sleep deprived.

We live in a sleep-deprived nation. The average adult only gets 6 hours of sleep per day when we should be getting 7 to 8 hours. Don't even get me going about children... Young children should get 10 to 11 hours per day and preteens and teens (12-18 years old), 8 ½ to 10 hours per day. Our kids are going to school sleep-deprived daily (this could be a separate chapter...or perhaps a book in itself). Sleep duration has decreased year by year in developed countries such as the U.S. How does all of this relate to obesity? Sleep affects our habits. Habits are our lifestyle. You choose to have a healthy lifestyle or a not-so-healthy lifestyle.

If you don't get enough sleep, you generally are not thinking clearly the next day. You may even be in a bad mood. Without adequate sleep, the last thing you would want to do is exercise, because you are tired. You may push yourself, which is great, but you won't exercise as hard and for the length of time you would have with the proper sleep. There are very few people who can function fine on six hours of sleep per day. In fact, researchers at the University of California discovered that some people (less than 3 percent of the population) have a gene that allows them to function fine (think clearly, make good decisions, etc.) with six hours or less of sleep per day. The rest of us (97% of population) need more than six hours and many of us simply are not getting it.

In the National Health and Nutrition Examination Study (NHANES1), inadequate sleep was considered a risk factor for obesity. This was published in a journal called *Sleep* in 2005. That's right, higher BMIs were directly associated with less sleep.

A study was carried out in Japan by Itani and colleagues in which shift workers (evening workers) were compared to non-shift workers. Less than 5 hours of sleep resulted in greater onset of obesity than those with 5 to 7 hours of sleep. The effects of shift work on sleep has received increased attention since shift work accounts for 20% of the entire workforce in developed countries.

A similar study by Niedhammer and colleagues looked at almost 500 nurses who worked the evening shift and reported an increased rate of obesity in these workers. This study, as well as another study by Mallon and colleagues, showed that there was also a higher incidence of diabetes and hypertension in individuals with short sleep duration. The problem with this, of course, is that obesity brings on these other problems, though the later study did try to control for existing obesity.

Who needs to look at recent studies when it happens to you? Years ago, before I read about any of these studies, I noticed the relationship between sleep and overeating. When I didn't sleep well, I ate more and exercised less. So I planned for this chapter many years ago, in fact, before I knew any studies existed. Take notice of whether lack of sleep affects your lifestyle in a negative way.

Let's say it does. Let's say that you do take notice and find that when you sleep less, you don't care about what you eat and you exercise less. What can you do to get to sleep an hour or two earlier? I have suggested one to two more hours of sleep for my patients and this has helped them with their weight loss efforts tremendously. They made better choices about food and definitely exercised more regularly.

Another thing you may want to take notice of is *what you are eating* in the early afternoon or in the evening. Some diet-related problems associated with sleep include drinking beverages with caffeine or eating foods very high in sodium. A surefire way to toss and turn at night is to have a cup of coffee at 3:00 p.m. when you are feeling that late afternoon "slump." Yes, it will give you a nice pick-me-up so that you can finish the work day and head home to your next set of responsibilities or your fun time, but that pick-me-up can cost you at the end of your evening.

Everyone reacts to caffeine differently. I know people who can drink a cup of coffee and go to bed and sleep like babies. Conversely, I know people (including myself) who cannot sleep at night even if that cup of coffee was in the afternoon. My advice to you: Know thyself. Take note of what happens when you've had coffee, tea, chocolate, or cola (particularly diet colas, which can be higher in caffeine than non-diet) in the late afternoon or evening. Think twice before ordering that espresso or cappuccino after dinner when you are out at a restaurant. This is where keeping a food log pays off. If you have written down what you ate and drank, you can refer back to this log and see if your lack of sleep corresponds to caffeine or another diet-related problem.

Aside from sleep, caffeine can also create problems for the person watching their weight because after caffeine's surge, the blood sugar drops, leaving one hungry. So while a cup of tea or coffee might help for the moment if you "want a little something," you will still "want a little something" later and it will be a physiological need at that moment, not your imagination.

In addition to caffeine, sodium is also another culprit in the sleep department. Many patients over the years have complained about not being able to sleep because they are very thirsty before bed. Did you ever have Chinese food, which is very high in sodium, and find yourself wide awake at night? How about hotdogs? Popcorn? OK, you get the idea. These are the foods you want to stay away from too late at night or at least go easy on (eat in small amounts) in the evening. I have listed the top twelve high-sodium foods to stay away from if salt affects your sleep (see side bar).

OK, I saved the obvious for last here: If you stay awake longer in the evening, what do you think you might do? *Eat*! Right? There is a reason for it so don't blame yourself. Your body is ready for another meal. Think about it. If your last meal was 6:30 p.m. and now it's 11:00 p.m.

Top Twelve High-Sodium Foods	
Food	Sodium content
TV Dinner	≥1150 mg
Packaged Food	
Chinese/Japanese (Ramen) noodles	1960 mg/pkg 1430 mg/C.
Mac & cheese (1 C)	≥ 580 mg
Canned Soup (1 C)	≥1000 mg
Chinese Food	
Beef & Broccoli (6 oz beef)	2400 mg
Egg drop/wonton soup (1 C)	850 mg
Hot Dogs (1)	900 mg
Microwave popcorn	>570 mg/3 C.
Teriyaki or soy sauce (1 tsp)	700-1000 mg
Tomato Juice (1 C)	650 mg
Spaghetti Sauce (1/2 C)	≥600 mg
Packaged Deli Meat (2 slices)	≥500 mg
Barbecue sauce or Catsup (1 Tbsp)	≥190 mg

or later, your food is digested. You may start to feel some emptiness in the ole stomach. That's a strong urge to ignore. If you are sleeping, it is definitely easier to ignore. The other thing that is hard to ignore late at night are the television commercials depicting food. How can you look at a sizzling hamburger being grilled right before your eyes when you ate over five hours ago? I, personally, cannot tell you how many times I have gone into the kitchen after seeing these commercials. Why do this to ourselves? Go to bed!

Now that you realize the connection between sleep and weight, you may want to try these suggestions if you need to obtain more sleep, but are having difficulty:

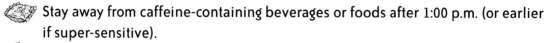 Stay away from caffeine-containing beverages or foods after 1:00 p.m. (or earlier if super-sensitive).

Do not eat high-sodium foods as a late dinner or evening snack.

Avoid exercise before bedtime. Try to get exercise earlier than three hours before bedtime. Exercise can be arousing and it decreases the secretion of melatonin, a natural tranquilizer.

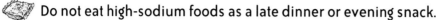 Avoid deep or critical thinking before bedtime. Such issues may affect your sleep because you may start worrying or thinking further about the issues.

If you are worrying or trying to remember something for the next day, write it down. You can refer to your note the next day.

Listen to soothing music.

Take a warm bath or shower to relax muscles. (Aromatherapy in the bath adds to the feeling of relaxation.)

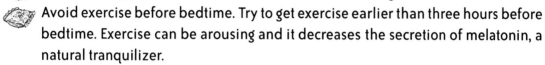 Turn off all electronics (computer, cell phone, television). In fact, for best sleep, these devices should not even be in the bedroom. A glaring computer light can easily keep one from sleeping. Light also decreases the production of melatonin. A TV left on by a spouse can affect your sleep (you may become interested in a program instead of falling asleep). These devices are not at all conducive to sleep.

If you need a snack, have a glass of low-fat milk or small bowl of low-sugar cereal with low-fat milk.

Wear comfortable, light-weight clothing. Avoid wearing heavy clothing such as flannels that can be too warm.

Set a good temperature for the room. If the temperature is too hot or too cold, you may have trouble falling asleep or wake up after a few hours.

Avoid naps during the day (or limit to a 20-minute power nap). Sleeping during the day interferes with the ability to get to sleep at a reasonable time in the evening.

Get into the habit of making your bed every day. It is more relaxing to get into a neatly made bed than to get into a bed with sheet and blankets pushed down to the foot of the bed.

Have a set bedtime each evening. Go to bed at the same time every night and wake up the same time, keeping weekends fairly close to weekdays.

Develop a bedtime routine. Establish a pattern of doing the same thing prior to bed each evening (ex. Read with a warm drink, meditate, pray.)

Like everything else in this book, I am recommending you add more sleep *gradually*. If you usually go to bed at 1:00 a.m., you may want to start going to bed at 11:30 p.m. or midnight. Do not try to go at 10:00 p.m. as it's too different from your previous habit. Eventually try to establish a bedtime that allows for a sleep that leaves you feeling refreshed in the morning and able to think clearly and make good decisions (and lifestyle choices). Hopefully some of the above ideas will be of help to those of you who are having trouble sleeping or those of you who go to bed too late and may have some difficulty establishing an earlier bedtime routine. Happy Sleeping! Remember sleep is critical to good health and a healthy weight.

PART FOUR:

Go for It!
(Application)

CHAPTER 10:

"1 Thing" Ideas: Better Food Choices

This chapter is divided into different categories for making changes in diet: Beverages, Snacks/Sweets, and Main Entrees. Included are calories saved each time you make the change and how much weight loss (theoretically) will occur each month and by one year. For just about every suggestion I make, I have an actual story that accompanies the suggestion, but I have chosen to share only those that are surprising or interesting.

I hope you can relate to one or two of these substitutions and find that it wouldn't take much work at all to make a change such as those below:

~~~~ Beverages ~~~~

Habit:
Coffee with cream (1/2 Tbsp) and 2 sugars (2 tsp)*
12 oz. cup *70 calories*

If you switch to:	Calories You will save:	In one month You will lose:	In one year You will lose:
Coffee with 2% milk & 1 sugar			
1/day	40	1/3 lb.	4.2 lbs.
2/day	80	2/3 lb.	8.4 lbs.
3/day	120	1 lb.	12.5 lbs.

Coffee with 2% milk, no sugar

1/day	55	½ lb.	5.7 lbs.
2/day	110	1 lb.	11.4 lbs.
3/day	160	1 ½ lb.	17.1 lbs.

Coffee – black

1/day	70	¾ lb.	7.3 lbs.
2/day	140	1 ¼ lbs.	14.6 lbs.
3/day	210	2 lbs.	21.9 lbs.

---

*Amazing: A coffee drinker who drinks 3 cups per day w/cream & sugar who switches to black will lose 22 pounds in one year!

Hot Cocoa
12 oz. cup *120 calories*

If you switch to:	Calories You will save:	In one month You will lose:	In one year You will lose:
Lite cocoa			
1/day	40	1/3 lb.	4.2 lbs.
2/day	80	2/3 lb.	8.4 lbs.
3/day	120	1 lb.	12.5 lbs.
Decaf flavored tea			
1/day	120	1 lb.	12.5 lbs.
2/day	240	2 lbs.	25 lbs.
3/day	360	3 lbs.	36 lbs.
Hot water*			
1/day	120	1 lb.	12.5 lbs.
2/day	240	2 lbs.	25 lbs.
3/day	360	3 lbs.	36 lbs.

*Actual Story: Many years ago, the office I worked at was repeatedly cold. A colleague and I found ourselves drinking hot cocoa (something supplied at the office) just to help keep warm. When we stopped to realize that the two hot cocoas we drank per day were adding up, we switched to plain hot water. Though I would love to take credit for this, it was actually my co-worker's idea (thanks, Maria, I still do this!). We didn't really want the hot cocoa, we wanted to be warm! The hot water did the trick just fine! We saved 5,160 calories per month (or 1.5 pounds per month) and 18 pounds per year!

Lemonade
12 oz. glass   *125 calories*

If you switch to:	Calories You will save:	In one month You will lose:	In one year You will lose:
Crystal Light® or			
Other sugar-free lemon drink			
1/day	125	1 lb.	13.0 lbs.
2/day	250	2 lbs.	26.1 lbs.
3/day	375	3 lbs.	39.1 lbs.
4/day	500	4 lbs.	52.1 lbs.

Iced Tea, sweetened
12 oz. glass   *130 calories*

If you switch to:	Calories You will save:	In one month You will lose:	In one year You will lose:
Crystal Light® Iced Tea or			
Other sugar-free iced tea drink			
1/day	130	1 lb.	13.6 lbs.

2/day	260	2 lbs.	27.2 lbs.
3/day	390	3 lbs.	40.8 lbs.
4/day	520	4 lbs.	54.2 lbs.

Soda
12 oz. can *150 calories*

If you switch to:	*Calories* *You will save:*	*In one month* *You will lose:*	*In one year* *You will lose:*
Diet Soda*			
1/day	150	1 1/3 lbs.	15.6 lbs.
2/day	300	2 2/3 lbs.	31.3 lbs.
3/day	450	4 lbs.	46.9 lbs.
4/day	600	5 1/3 lbs.	62.5 lbs.

---

*Actual Story: I've already told you about Beverly (Chapter 1) who lost 14 pounds in 3 months after switching from regular Coke to Diet Coke and Fresca. Theoretically, my chart shows 4 pounds per month (or 12 pounds in 3 months). Beverly lost a few more pounds than this.

If you are still drinking regular soda, consider the diet version or seltzer water instead. This has been done with hundreds of patients over the years who have been happy with their weight loss and feel it was a minimal change. I forgot to mention that once you switch to diet soda, there's no going back!

Soda
20 oz. bottle *250 calories*

While writing this book, the typical size of a soda increased. In many stores, you cannot purchase a can of soda, but must purchase a 20-oz. bottle. Interestingly enough, the can is already 4 oz. more than a "serving size" or 1.5 servings, but now the bottle is 2.5 servings! Unfortunately, most people drink the entire bottle.

If you are wondering why people are getting heavier and heavier over the years and why the rates of obesity are climbing, look at how the serving sizes of foods have increased over the years. We grow according to the serving sizes available.

If you switch to:	Calories You will save:	In one month You will lose:	In one year You will lose:
Diet Soda (20 oz. bottle)			
1/day	250	2 lbs.	25.7 lbs.
2/day	500	4 lbs..	51.4 lbs.
3/day	750	6 lbs.	77.1 lbs.

Fruit Punch or Fruit Juice
12 oz. glass *180 calories*

If you switch to:	Calories You will save:	In one month You will lose:	In one year You will lose:
Crystal Light® Raspberry Ice or Other sugar-free fruit-flavored drink			
1/day	180	1.6 lbs.	18.8 lbs.
2/day	360	3.2 lbs.	37.5 lbs.
3/day	540	4.8 lbs.	56.3 lbs.
4/day	720	6.4 lbs.	75.1 lbs.

Whole Milk
8 oz.   *150 calories*

If you switch to:	Calories You will save:	In one month You will lose:	In one year You will lose:
2% Milk			
1/day	30	.27 lbs.	3.1 lbs.
2/day	60	.53 lbs.	6.3 lbs.
3/day	90	.80 lbs.	9.4 lbs.
1% Milk			
1/day	50	.44 lbs.	5.2 lbs.
2/day	100.	.88 lbs.	10.4 lbs.
3/day	150	1.3 lbs.	15.6 lbs.
Skim Milk			
1/day	60	.5 lbs.	6.3 lbs.
2/day	120.	1.1 lbs.	12.6 lbs.
3/day	180	1.6 lbs.	18.8 lbs.

Wine
6 oz. glass *120 calories*

If you switch to:	Calories You will save:	In one month You will lose:	In one year You will lose:
Wine Spritzer			
(1/2 wine, ½ seltzer)			
1/day	60	.5 lbs.	6.3 lbs.
2/day	120	1.1 lbs.	12.5 lbs.
Seltzer			
1/day	120	1.1 lbs.	12.5 lbs.
2/day	240	2.1 lbs.	25.0 lbs.

Beer
12 oz. can *140 calories*

If you switch to:	Calories You will save:	In one month You will lose:	In one year You will lose:
Light version			
1/day	40	.3 lb.	4.2 lbs.
2/day	80	.7 lb.	8.4 lbs.
Seltzer w/fresh lemon or lime			
1/day	140	1.2 lbs.	14.6 lbs.
2/day	280	2.4 lbs.	29.2 lbs.

Martini
3 oz. cocktail *185 calories*

If you switch to:	Calories You will save:	In one month You will lose:	In one year You will lose:
Seltzer w/fresh lemon or lime			
1/day	185	1.6 lbs.	19.3 lbs.
2/day	370	3.3 lbs.	38.6 lbs.
Gingerale, regular (12 oz.)			
1/day	65	.6 lbs.	6.8 lbs.
2/day	130	1.2 lbs.	13.6 lbs.
Tomato Juice (Virgin Bloody Mary), 6 oz.			
1/day	150	1.3 lbs.	15.6 lbs.
2/day	300	2.7 lbs.	31.3 lbs.

~~~~ Snacks/Sweets ~~~~

Peanuts
Dry roasted, 1.1 oz. snack bag   *195 calories*

If you switch to:	Calories You will save:	In one month You will lose:	In one year You will lose:
Pretzels* (.5 oz. snack bag)	145	1.3 lbs.	15.1 lbs.

---

*Actual Story: A man whom I know took the train home from New York to Connecticut Monday through Friday. He would eat a snack bag of peanuts on the way home every day. He switched to a snack bag of pretzels (33 mini) and lost 15 pounds in one year with this one change (and he only did this five days a week!).

Switching from potato chips to popcorn (below) makes an even bigger difference!

Potato Chips   *320 calories*
2 oz.

If you switch to:	Calories You will save:	In one month You will lose:	In one year You will lose:
Popcorn, lite (3 C.)	240	2.1 lbs.	25.2 lbs.

Cheese & Crackers
(2 oz. Cheese, 6 crackers)   *310 calories*

If you switch to:	Calories You will save:	In one month You will lose:	In one year You will lose:
Assorted olives (10 large)			
Italian bread (1 oz.)			
Olive oil (1 tsp)	110	1.1 lbs.	11.5 lbs.
Vegetables & Dip			
Celery (2 stalks)			
Carrots (3 oz.)			
Ranch Dip (low fat, 1 Tbsp)	170	1.5 lbs.	17.8 lbs.

Ice Cream, Chocolate
1 C.   *465 calories*

If you switch to:	Calories You will save:	In one month You will lose:	In one year You will lose:
Frozen Yogurt, Chocolate (1 C.)	240	2.1 lbs.	25.2 lbs.
Fudgesicle* (1 pop)	430	3.8 lbs.	44.8 lbs.

---

*Amazing: A daily ice cream consumer could really save pounds by switching to fudgesicles—45 pounds in one year...what a lick'n on the pounds!

Vanilla Sandwich Cookies
(2 Cookies) *120 calories*

If you switch to:	Calories You will save:	In one month You will lose:	In one year You will lose:
Nilla Wafers (4 Cookies)	50	.4 lbs.	5.2 lbs.
Animal Crackers (4 Cookies)	76	.7 lbs.	8.0 lbs.

Apple Pie
(1/8 frozen pie) *230 Calories*

If you switch to:	Calories You will save:	In one month You will lose:	In one year You will lose:
Baked Apple (Medium, with cinnamon)	140	1.3 lbs.	14.6 lbs.

~~~~Main Entrees ~~~~

Big Mac
Large Fries
Regular Coke (24 oz.) *1430 Calories*

If you switch to:	Calories You will save:	In one month You will lose:	In one year You will lose:
Grilled Chicken Sandwich or Regular-sized hamburger Small Fries Diet Coke	960	8.3 lbs.	100.1 lbs.

More realistically, if you switch once per week, at the end of the year you will lose 14.3 lbs.

Amazing: I don't know anyone who actually made this change daily, but if you have seen the movie *Supersize Me*, you have seen that the actor gained 30 pounds in one month from eating all three meals per day at McDonald's. My realistic recommendation is to change to a better choice if you eat at a fast-food establishment at least once per day (or whenever you do). This change daily would potentially lead to an 8-pound or more weight loss in just one month!

Fried Fish Platter   *1050 calories*
(Fried shrimp and/or scallops with fries and coleslaw)
6-8 large shrimp, 6-8 large scallops, tartar sauce (2 T), lemon,
Fries (20 pcs), and coleslaw (1/2 C)

If you switch to:	Calories	In one month	In one year
	You will save:	You will lose:	You will lose:
Broiled Fish Dinner	675	6 lbs.	70.4 lbs.

(Broiled shrimp and/or scallops with baked potato and green beans)
6-8 large shrimp (3 oz.), 6-8 large scallops (3 oz), lemon,
Baked potato (medium to large), sour cream (1 T) or butter (1 tsp),
Steamed green beans (1/2 C)

More realistically, if you switch once per week, at the end of the year, you will lose 10 lbs.

Mozzarella & Sausage/Pepperoni Pizza, Regular crust
(2 pcs)   *700 calories*

If you switch to:	*Calories You will save:*	*In one month You will lose:*	*In one year You will lose:*
Mozzarella & Fresh Tomato, or Vegetables, Thin crust (2 pcs)	300	2.6 lbs.	31.3 lbs.

More realistically, if you switch once per week, at the end of the year, you will lose 4.5 lbs.

"Easy" on the mozzarella with Fresh Tomato or Vegetables, Thin crust (2 pcs)	400	3.5 lbs.	41.7 lbs.

More realistically, if you switch once per week, at the end of the year, you will lose 6 lbs.

Amazing: The easiest way to cut calories from your pizza is to blot it before eating it. Yes, I said blot it! Just like blotting lipstick, you should blot your pizza. Flip it over on the paper plate to absorb some of the oil or simply take a paper towel and press down lightly on the pizza before eating it. Check out the grease on the plate or your paper towel!

If you like oil on the pizza, you may want to order a thin crust pizza to save calories. You save 60-70 calories per slice by ordering a thin crust. I like regular crust, not too thin. I'd rather blot than give up my crust!

Obviously adding meats as a topping versus vegetables is going to be higher in calories. The meat is much higher in fat, which is why the calorie level rises. If you don't want to give up your meat, you may want to order a mix of vegetable and meat (sausage and spinach, for example).

Buono Appetito!

General Tsao's Chicken (4 oz. chicken)
w/rice (1 C)   *950 calories*

If you switch to:	*Calories*	*In one month*	*In one year*
	You will save:	*You will lose:*	*You will lose:*
Chicken and broccoli			
(4 oz. chicken w/2 C broccoli)			
w/rice (1 C)	320	2.8 lbs.	33.4 lbs.

More realistically, if you switch once per week, at the end of the year, you will lose 4.8 lbs.

Bologna or Salami (2 slices)
And Cheese (2 slices) Sandwich
w/mayonnaise (2 tsp)   *635 calories*

If you switch to:	*Calories*	*In one month*	*In one year*
	You will save:	*You will lose:*	*You will lose:*
Turkey or chicken (2 slices)			
And Cheese (1 slice) Sandwich			
w/mustard	265	2.3 lbs.	27.3 lbs.
or			
Lean Roast Beef or Ham (2 slices)			
And Cheese (1 slice) Sandwich			
w/mustard	225	1.9 lbs.	23.1 lbs.

Hopefully you found a substitution for a habit you are currently doing. Be patient with yourself. Every calorie, literally, *does* count long term. Remember: every extra 3500 calories ingested turns into fat. You can do the math. If you take in 200 calories less than before every day (by changing a food choice), 200 X number of days you made the change = total calories saved. Lastly, divide calories saved by 3500 to see how many pounds you could lose with the change. So the formula is:

Calories Saved in One Sitting X Number of Days Normally Consumed = Total Calories Saved

Total Calories Saved/3500 = Number of Pounds To be Lost With the Change During Days Normally Consumed
Multiply by Number of months if you are looking for a yearly estimated weight loss.

Let's take the 200 calories from above:
200 X 30 days (let's say you make a change that effects you every day of the month) = 6000 calories saved.
6000/3500 = 1.71 pounds to be lost that month!

Now take the 1.71 pounds and multiply by 12 for the amount you would lose if you did this for entire year:

1.71 pounds X 12 = 20.5 pounds lost per year!!

If you cannot find something that relates to you, write down what you eat each day and pinpoint the high-calorie culprit. Ask for help from a dietitian or find a substitution in a calorie publication. Most of these calorie totals were derived from a book called *Bowes & Church's Food Values of Portions Commonly Used* (J. A. . Pennington and J. Spungen, 2010). This book is a dietitian's lifeline, but anyone can learn how to use it fairly quickly for food comparison purposes. There are also several websites or apps that calculate calories.

In Appendix B.1, "What's Your One Thing?", you will find a worksheet to list your idea, how many calories you will save with your idea, and how much weight loss you have seen with it.

In the next chapter we will use the same idea of saving calories, but relate it to exercise. Instead of saving calories, we will estimate how many calories have been expended (burned).

CHAPTER 11:

"1 Thing" Ideas: More Activity

Now that you know many of the benefits obtained from activity, here are some suggestions about ways to get regular exercise and how many calories would be burned, along with how many pounds you would lose from these expended calories.

The number of calories you burn depends on three factors: the exercise you do, your weight, and the time spent engaging in the exercise. Some exercises are clearly more strenuous than others. The more your heart and muscles work, the more the body calls for energy. The more you weigh, the more calories you will burn. The estimations below were all based on an individual weighing 180 pounds. If a person were to weigh just 20 pounds more, the calories burned would jump to about 15% more calories expended. The extra weight is acting like resistance, calling for more energy expenditure. Lastly, the more time you engage in an activity, the more calories you burn.

Whether you are able to walk a treadmill one hour per day or simply take a short walk outdoors (like Mrs. Cunningham at the beginning of the book), there will probably be some scenario here that you could apply to your daily regimen.

Adding Habits to Your Daily Routine:

New Habit:	Min/Day:	Calories You will burn:	In one month You will lose:	In one year You will lose:
Walking Dog	20	76	.66 lbs.	7.8 lbs.
Walking Moderately	20	82	.70 lbs.	8.4 lbs.
Walking Moderately	45	180	1.5 lbs.	18.5 lbs.
Walking on treadmill, briskly	20	92	.80 lbs.	9.5 lbs.

---

*Actual Story: As I have mentioned earlier, when I was young I worked in a commercial weight loss industry. One of my jobs was to weigh individuals each week and set goals with them so that they could achieve a weight loss the following week. One of my clients, Mrs. Cunningham, who was extremely sedentary, started walking to the mailbox each day and then down the street, to eventually a mile a day. Before she even started with a distance of a mile a day, I saw a drop in the scale after months of maintaining her weight with diet alone. As stated in Chapter 1, this 62-year-old woman lost 20 pounds by adding regular walking to her regimen.

Dancing	20	136	1.2 lbs.	14.0 lbs.
Dancing	30	204	1.8 lbs.	21.0 lbs.
Stretching/Yoga	30	115	1.0 lbs.	12.0 lbs.
Calisthetics	20	95	.82 lbs.	9.8 lbs.
Jump Rope, Moderately	10	136	1.2 lbs.	14.0 lbs.
Biking, light (10-11.9 mph)	20	163	1.4 lbs.	16.8 lbs.
Biking. moderately (10-11.9 mph)	30	245	2.1 lbs.	25.2 lbs.
Rowing Machine, Light	20	191	1.6 lbs.	19.6 lbs.

Rowing Machine, Moderately	30	286	2.45 lbs.	29.4 lbs.
Running 12 min. mile	12	131	1.1 lbs.	13.2 lbs.
Running/Jogging on Treadmill, moderately	30	239	2.1	25.2 lbs.
Swimming Free style, slow	20	191	1.6 lbs.	19.6 lbs.

*Actual Story: Recently a patient of mine lost 17 pounds buying groceries! Actually, she walked to the store every single day for almost 6 months and purchased only one or two items. She lives about a mile from the store on a main road. Instead of driving to the store and buying 15 items all at once, she decided that she would walk with a destination.

Originally, I laughed at this idea, but it's actually very creative. There is not a day that goes by that my patients do not teach me something!

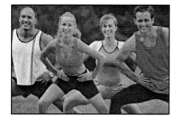

Adding Habits 2 or 3 Times Per Week

Exercise Class at Gym	1 hr., 3 X/wk	531 each time X 3	2.0 lbs.	24.0 lbs.
Health Club Exercise (1/2 cardio, 1/2 weights)	1 hr. 3 X/wk	449 each time X 3	1.7 lbs.	20.0 lbs.
Kickboxing Class	1 hr., 3 X/wk	817 each time X 3	3.0 lbs.	36.0 lbs.
Basketball Non-game	1 hr., 2 X/wk	490 each time X 2	1.2 lbs.	14.5 lbs.
Dance Class, Ballroom Moderately fast	1 hr., 2 X/wk	449 each time X 2	1.1 lbs.	13.2 lbs.
Hiking	1.5 hrs., 2 X/wk	735 each time X 2	1.8 lbs.	21.7 lbs.

Hiking with

5-8 lbs on back   1.5 hrs., 2 X/wk   873 each time X 2   2.1 lbs.   25.7 lbs.

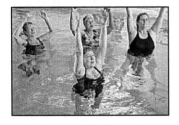

If you recall earlier, I stated the more you weigh, the more calories you burn. When you add weight to your routine (carrying weights, for example), this is similar to weighing more while exercising.

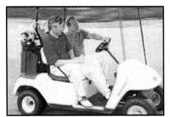

Golfing*,

Using Cart   2 hrs., 1 X/wk   572 each time X 1   .7 lbs.   8.5 lbs.

---

*Lighten Things Up:

Ok, let's be serious here. You'll want to go for a beer after the golf game. You're thinking, "Well, I'll put back all the calories I took off." Guess what? It's still worth it and the truth is you *won't* pack the calories on that you've just burned. If you order a lite beer (which many people do, anyway) at 95 calories, you would have burned 477 calories for the 2-hour game vs 572. This still equates to 2/3 pound per month or 7 pounds at the end of one year! Not too bad for having a good time!

Golfing,
Walking and pulling clubs   2 hrs, 1 X/wk   702 each time X 1   .9 lbs.   10.3 lbs

Some of the above activities may be considered structured in nature. Walking the dog might be more "here and there" however. This chapter would not be complete if lower intensity or shorter bursts of activities were not available to those who don't like to work

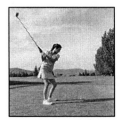

out or simply can only obtain activities in their regular day routine of work and caring for children.

Regular Habit:	Min/Day:	Calories You will burn:	In one month You will lose:	In one year You will lose:
Walking moderately from car to work, Then work to car (assumes work 5 days/ wk)	5 min. ea. time	44	.27 lbs.	3.2 lbs.
Playing with kids	15	85	.73 lbs.	8.7 lbs.
Playing Tag with kids (assumes 3 1-min breaks)	15	130	1.1 lbs.	13.4 lbs.
Pre-shower Workout* (Takes less than 5 minutes)	<5 min.	47	.40 lbs.	4.8 lbs.

**10 head rolls (5 each direction), 20 shoulder rolls (backwards), 2 deep breaths extending arms up and down, 40 stretches to the ceiling followed by 100 jumping jacks, ending with 5 deep breaths for a "cool down." This literally takes five minutes or less of your time before getting into the shower.

Playing with your Kids

There is certainly something to be said for playing with your children. It may sound silly, but try it. The first time I played tag with my son several years ago, I felt like a kid again. It was invigorating. Perhaps the more important benefit here is that your children will love it!! They will love the fact that *you* are playing with them. You will be bonding with your child while getting necessary exercise.

Our children are losing out on the act of playing. Television and video and computer games have taken the place of free play in our society. What happened to good old-fashioned, creative fun! It's free and it's healthy!

The obesity rate for both adults and children has sky rocketed over the past few decades. Although there are several contributors to childhood obesity, the lack of outside play has played a tremendous role. Technology certainly has its pros, but overall our children are suffering from the sedentary lifestyles they are living today.

Get out and play with your child!!...even if for only 15 minutes per day!!

This chapter could be 100 pages long. There are so many ways to become more active! I hope you found at least one or two ideas that you could apply to your daily or weekly routine. In Appendix B.2, "What's Your One Thing?" you will find a worksheet to list the "thing" you determined to do differently to increase your activity level.

The next chapter, "Becoming More Aware," may help you determine where in your day you could find time to exercise. Becoming aware of your lifestyle is the key that "opens the door" to making changes.

CHAPTER 12:

Becoming More Aware

The man who is aware of himself is henceforward independent...
~~President Richard M. Nixon

This is perhaps the most important chapter in this book (besides Chapters 10 and 11, which actually give ideas about making small changes that elicit significant results). Why is this chapter so critical? Because awareness, coupled with a bit of motivation, is the 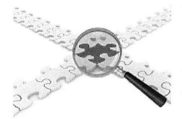 first step to change in our behavior. How can we modify our current, destructive pattern if we don't know what to change? Incidentally, I am not referring to changing the type of foods we eat. I am talking about changing how we act—changing what is familiar to us and feeling awkward, wracked, or irritated. Trying to figure out what your triggers are or what your high-risk situations are is work! More work than going on a diet, which is short-term. It is easier to decide that you are going to eat cabbage, steak, or grapefruit for the next seven days, than it is to learn "what's eating you" and what you should do about it.

Behavior that results in overeating is like a chain or a staircase. One event leads to the next. In order to have a chain, you have several links and in order to walk up the stairs, you have several steps which you must take. Behavior that makes it easier to trigger overeating can be referred to as a "weak link" or a "faulty step." A simple example is in order: If John loved cookies and found himself eating a bunch of them every night at 10:00 p.m., do you think John should keep cookies in his cabinets? The "faulty step" would be buying the cookies. He will never "make it up the steps" if he buys cookies and is not sleeping by 10:00 p.m. Another example of "taking a flop" would be Sally buying soda for her children when she loves it herself. If Sally doesn't choose something different for her children to drink at home, she will constantly be faced with a high-risk situation of pouring soda for her children.

Sometimes examples are not as clear as those suggested above. Let's look at one that requires more insight: Raymond has not been getting along with his wife for months. They have two small children that require a lot of work, as most children do. Raymond comes home from work 7:00 p.m. or later most nights. His job is demanding so he eats very little lunch on the run, if any. When he gets home at 7:00 p.m., the first thing he does is eat because he is famished. He spends very little time with the children, which his wife resents. Some evenings the children are already bathed and Raymond simply reads them a bedtime story after eating his dinner. As you can imagine, his wife is exhausted. She works full-time, brings the children to and from daycare, and is the primary caregiver of the children. A typical evening for Raymond is sitting in front of the TV and snacking because he wants to avoid the usual argument with his wife. Raymond is 60 pounds overweight and is inquiring about the XYZ diet. Do you think he should go on it?

Hopefully, you said no to Raymond about going on the XYZ diet. My next question: What are the faulty steps or weak links to the above scenario? The first and foremost is eating a small lunch or skipping it completely. It is possible that working until 7:00 p.m. is an additional weak link but only if Raymond has any control over this (Does he come home at 7:00 p.m. intentionally or does his company require him to work this late?). Eating lunch would allow him to interact with his wife and children for a few minutes when he got home instead of eating right away because he is famished. Perhaps he could bathe the children, eat dinner, and then read them a bedtime story. His wife might not be as upset since he took on an extra responsibility. This would, of course, lead to improved communication between him and his wife and a possible pleasant evening shared with his wife (and not the TV). It is my guess that he would eat a smaller dinner, overall, since he is not as hungry as he was when he skipped lunch and he would have a much smaller snack in the evening because he isn't sitting in front of the TV for hours, unaware of the calories taken in and finding comfort in the food he's eating. All of this adds up to less calories. How would Raymond learn what his high-risk situation was if he didn't have the help of someone pointing it out to him? This is where the importance of diaries comes into play. I will share two different types with you.

The first is more comprehensive (food and mood journal) while the second (steps to success) is simply a snapshot of a situation. You may need to fill out several copies of the second method in order to become more aware of why you are overeating.

Food, Mood and Activity Record

This is an expanded food diary because it includes what mood you were in before or during eating, who you were with, where you were, and how hungry you were. It also includes an area to fill in any physical activity you had, because this can play a role in eating more or less as well.

FOOD, MOOD AND ACTIVITY RECORD

Name:_____   Date:_____

TIME	PLACE Home, friend"s house, or restaurant	FOOD Describe in detail, include brand names, how food was cooked, etc.	HOW MUCH FOOD Teaspoon, ounces or cups	HUNGER Scale 1-5 1=not hungry 5=starving	FEELINGS Sad, angry, bored, happy, lonely, etc.	PLANNED OR "HERE AND THERE" Or SEDENTARY ACTIVITIES What activity, how many, how long

Time. It is best to fill this in throughout the day so that you don't forget situations in which you ate. You will also have difficulty recalling the quantity of food if you do not record right away. If you do not fill it in throughout the day, estimate the time of day you ate later when you have the Time to complete the Food, Mood and Activity Record.

Place. Were you at work, home, a friend's, or a restaurant? Where exactly were you when you ate?

Food. Describe the food you ate in detail. How was it prepared? What brand name was it? If it was milk, please describe what percent fat (skim, 1%, 2%, or whole). If it was hamburger meat or another type of beef, for example, try to explain its fat content (or indicate if it was a lean cut).

Quantity of Food. Be specific about the amount of food you ate. How many ounces, cups, tablespoons, or teaspoons? Try to estimate the cooked portion (not raw). If you don't know the exact amount you may want to use visual items such as the following to help you estimate:

1 cup = the size of a tennis ball.
½ cup = the size of a level ice cream scoop.
3 ounces (one suggested serving of meat or fish, for example) is the size of a deck of cards, cassette tape, or palm of your hand.
1 ounce = the size of your thumb.
1 tablespoon = the size of your thumb.
1 teaspoon = the size of your thumb tip.
1 ounce of cheese = the same size as a pair of dice.
One medium fruit or medium potato is about the same size as your fist or a tennis ball.

You may want to purchase a plastic set of measuring cups and spoons. It is not necessary, however, to purchase a food scale. Visualizing a deck of cards or cassette tape is good enough unless you are on a therapeutic diet for health purposes that restricts protein (in this case it would be wise to be most accurate).

I am sure you can appreciate why it is important to write in the journal directly after you eat. Portions may be much harder to recall later.

Degree of Hunger. Try to assess your level of hunger using a scale from 1-5. One refers to not being hungry at all and 5 refers to being famished. Again, I am sure you can appreciate the importance of completing this journal throughout the day rather than at the end of the day as it may be hard to try to recall how hungry you were at each meal or snack time.

Feelings. We eat in response to many feelings. Try to label how you are feeling when you eat. Boredom is a common emotion that accompanies snacking. Other feelings may be sad, angry, happy, lonely, disappointed, lazy, tired. We often eat when we are procrastinating from completing a project or a difficult task. Even if your journal is not handy, try labeling how you are feeling when you eat. This is a necessary skill to master when trying to become aware of eating triggers and to better manage your weight.

Activity. Recording activities have two benefits: (1) It may help you actually *do* an activity if you know you are expected to record such information, and (2) it enables you to look back and determine if physical activity helps you to eat less throughout the day. Try exercise at different times of the day to reveal if less consumption occurs daily as a result of physical activity.

Make several photocopies of the previous page or purchase a notebook and include all of the above elements. You will appreciate the detail you use later. More detail means greater insight later.

It is unrealistic to expect yourself to use a food diary *every* day. Life is far too busy to allow this. Three or four days per week is usually sufficient to find trends in your behavior. It is best to record at least one weekend day, as we typically eat very differently on the weekend than we do on a weekday. The remaining days should include at least two weekdays that are consecutive (any two weekdays as long as you do not skip a day in between). For example, if you decided to keep a food diary three days per week, Saturday, Tuesday, and Wednesday would be a great idea. If you decided to keep a food diary four days per week, Saturday, Monday, Tuesday, and Thursday would be fine.

Cindy kept the following food diary for three days. I'll fill you in about Cindy a bit and then ask you what we can learn from her food diaries. Cindy is a 27-year-old full-time high school English teacher. She is also taking one course in the evening at college to become a better public speaker. Typically she gets home from work at 4:00 p.m., walks the dog, prepares dinner, and watches the news. After that she settles down to correcting homework, tests, and papers or doing her own college homework.

Here are Cindy's food diaries:

FOOD, MOOD AND ACTIVITY RECORD

Name:___Cindy_____ Date:_____Day One, Tuesday_____

TIME	PLACE Home, friend"s house, or restaurant	FOOD Describe in detail, include brand names, how food was cooked, etc.	HOW MUCH FOOD Teaspoon, ounces or cups	HUNGER Scale 1-5 1=not hungry 5=starving	FEELINGS Sad, angry, bored, happy, lonely, etc.	PLANNED OR "HERE AND THERE" EXERCISE Or SEDENTARY ACTIVITIES What activity, how many, how long
6:15 am	home	Coffee w/ Sugar	1 C, 1 tsp.	3	tired	Woke up, show-ered
		Honey nut Cheerios	1 ½ C			
		Milk, 2%	1 C			
6:45 am	home					Let dog out; dress for work; leave
11:30 am	work	Ham American Cheese Bread, wheat Mayo Let & Tom Potato chips Diet soda	2 oz. 1 oz. 2 slices 1 Tbsp. Leaf/slice 2 handfuls 1 Can	5	Rushed, stressed	
3:00 pm	work	Granola bar Diet soda	1 1 Can	4	stressed	Planned next day lessons
4:15 pm	home					Walked dog 20 min.
5 pm	home					Watched news
						Prepared dinner

5:30 pm	home	Pasta Sauce Salad: lettuce,tomato Dressing, Ranch Bread, Italian Butter Parm cheese Diet soda	2 Cups ¾ Cup 2 Cups 2 Tbsp. 2 1" slices 2 tsp. 1 tsp 1 Can	4	Relaxing	
6 pm					Relaxing	Washed dishes, Cleaned up
6:30 pm					bored	Organized papers to correct, etc.;played with dog
6:45 pm		Chocolate kisses	10	1	bored	Getting ready to correct papers
						Turned TV on; surfed channels
7:15 pm		Hot Chocolate	1 C.	1	Bored, unmotivated	Talked on phone
7:45 pm		English Muffin Butter Jelly	1 1 Tbsp. 2 tsp.	2	tired	Getting ready To correct papers; correcting papers
8:30 pm		Coffee w/ sugar	1 C. 1 tsp.		Tired/bored	Correcting papers
9:15 pm		Coffee cake	2 indiv. wrapped		happy	Break from papers
9:30 pm					depressed	Finishing up papers
10 pm					relaxed	Watching TV
11 pm					tired	Went to bed

FOOD, MOOD AND ACTIVITY RECORD

Name: ____Cindy_____   Date: ____Day Two, Wednesday_____

TIME	PLACE Home, friend''s house, or restaurant	FOOD Describe in detail, include brand names, how food was cooked, etc.	HOW MUCH FOOD Teaspoon, ounces or cups	HUNGER Scale 1-5 1=not hungry 5=starving	FEELINGS Sad, angry, bored, happy, lonely, etc.	PLANNED OR "HERE AND THERE" EXERCISE Or SEDENTARY ACTIVITIES What activity, how many, how long
6:15 am	home	Coffee w/ Sugar	1 C, 1 tsp.	3	tired	Woke up, showered
		Honey nut Cheerios	1 ½ C			
		Milk, 2%	1 C			
6:45	home					Let dog out; dress for work; leave
11:30 am	work	Tuna American Cheese Bread, wheat Mayo Let & Tom Yogurt Diet soda	½ can 1 oz. 2 slices 1 Tbsp Leaf/slice 6 oz. 1 Can	5	Rushed, stressed	
3:15 pm	work	Granola bar Diet soda	2 1 Can	4	stressed	Planned next day lessons
4:30 pm	home					Walked dog 15 min.
5 pm	home					Watched news; Talked on phone
5:30 pm	home			4	Relaxed	Prepared dinner

6 pm	home	burger American cheese Roll catsup Salad: lettuce, tomato dressing, Ranch Diet soda	4 oz. 2 oz. 1 whole 2 Tbsp. 2 C. 2 Tbsp. 1 Can	4	Relaxed	
6:30 pm					bored	Washed dishes, cleaned up; washed clothes
7 pm					bored	Getting ready to finish writing own paper— due tomorrow!
7:15 pm		Chocolate kisses	8	1	bored	Talked on phone
7:45 pm					anxious	Writing paper
8pm		Potato chips	2 handfuls	1	anxious	Writing paper
8:30 pm		Hot chocolate	1 C.	1	Chilly, anx-ious	Writing paper
9 pm		Coffee cake	2 indiv. wrapped	1	tired	Writing paper
9:30 pm		Chocolate kisses	6	1	tired	Taking break; surfing channels
10:15 pm		French bread pizza Diet soda	1 1 can	3	Tired, bored	Finishing paper
11:15 pm					Very tired	Went to bed

FOOD, MOOD AND ACTIVITY RECORD

Name: Cindy   Date: Day Three, Saturday

TIME	PLACE Home, friend"s house, or restaurant	FOOD Describe in detail, include brand names, how food was cooked, etc.	HOW MUCH FOOD Teaspoon, ounces or cups	HUNGER Scale 1-5 1=not hungry 5=starving	FEELINGS Sad, angry, bored, happy, lonely, etc.	PLANNED OR "HERE AND THERE" EXERCISE Or SEDENTARY ACTIVITIES What activity, how many, how long
8:15 am	home				sleepy	Walked dog for 10 minutes
8:30 am	home	Coffee w/ Sugar	2 C. 2 tsp.	3	happy	ate; cleaned house for 1 hr.
		Honey nut Cheerios	1 ½ C.			
		Milk, 2%	1 C.			
10 am	gym	water	½ bottle			Met friend at Zumba class 1 hr.
11:30	home	water	½ bottle			Showered; got dressed; washed clothes
1 pm	Grocery store	grapes	10	4		Went food shopping 1 hr.
2:15 pm	Fast food	Grilled chicken sandwich French fries Diet soda	1 sandwich Medium 16 oz.	5		Ate in car in parking lot
2:30 pm	Driving					Finished Errands
3:30 pm	home	grapes	8			Put groceries away; talked on phone
5 pm	home					Took nap
6:30 pm						Took dog for walk 20 minutes; got ready to go out
7:30 pm	Restaurant	Wine Pizza, pepperoni	6 oz. 2 slices	5	Relaxed, happy	With a friend

9:15 pm	Movie theatre	Popcorn w/butter diet soda	2 C. 1 Tbsp. 24 oz.	1	Happy, a little tired	With a friend
11:30 pm	home				Very tired	Went to bed
11:45 pm		Orange juice	16 oz.	1	Can't sleep, very thirsty	

Where do we begin with Cindy's food records? There are so many ways to interpret them. We could comment on her food choices, but she started each day with good intentions and this continued, for the most part, through lunch. Yes, she had sweetened cereal at breakfast and her milk could have been lower in fat. Yes, she had potato chips once at lunch. These choices, however, were not her problem.

Did you notice a pattern about Cindy on the weekdays? What happened to Cindy when she got home from work? She ate dinner, watched the news, and got right to work... or did she? Cindy was a procrastinator. She turned to food instead of getting the job done. Two behaviors could have helped Cindy tremendously and she would have had to experiment with each one. She could have done something more active than walk the dog for 15 or 20 minutes when she got home. Maybe this would have broken her day up more so she wasn't leaving one job to go to the next (her own homework or correcting papers). This would have allowed her to relieve some anxiety and, perhaps, feel a bit more in control.

Cindy's other alternative would be to leave her house while writing a paper or correcting papers. When one turns to food during procrastination, you are better off in an area where there is no access to food. Perhaps the library would be a good place for Cindy to concentrate on her own writing so that she couldn't stop to look in the cabinets or to cook something.

Cindy is an emotional eater. She eats in response to boredom, stress, and anxiety. Overall, she seemed to do better when there was less stress. Her food choices were not very good on the weekend, but her portions were appropriate and she did not seem to be eating in response to anything but maybe the movie when she ordered the popcorn!

Steps to Success

As an alternative or change of pace to the food record, is my "Steps to Success" method. The idea of this is to write down the events that lead up to overeating. Start at the bottom and work your way up by writing down each event that occurred just before the overeating.

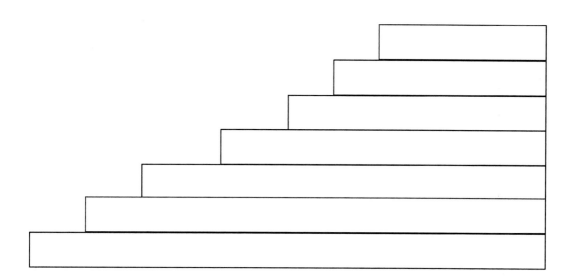

Let's take the example of Raymond from the beginning of the chapter. His staircase of events would look something like this:

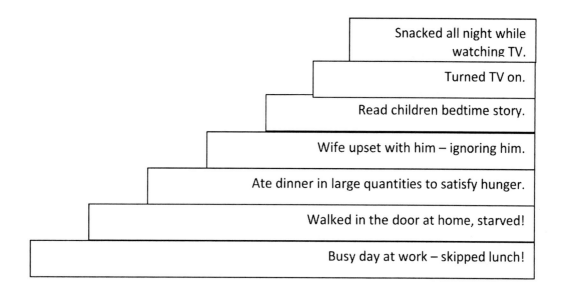

Snacked all night while watching TV.

Turned TV on.

Read children bedtime story.

Wife upset with him – ignoring him.

Ate dinner in large quantities to satisfy hunger.

Walked in the door at home, starved!

Busy day at work – skipped lunch!

After he analyzed his actions, his steps to success might look similar to this:

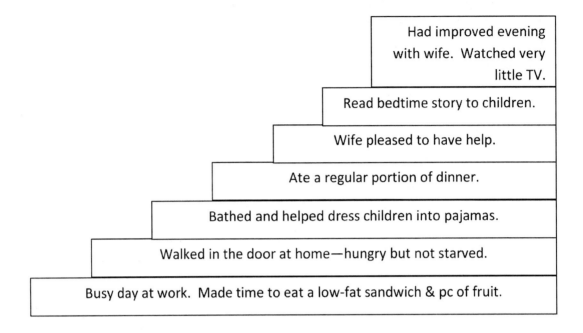

It is critical to identify the situation when you are most likely to overeat. Ask yourself the following questions: Who, What, Where, and When?

Who: Is it when you are with a certain person?

When I was younger, I tended to overeat with a particular friend. Whenever I went to the donut shop, I was always with the same friend.

When: Is it a certain time of the day?

Many people do their overeating in the evening. Pay attention to what you are doing while you overeat at this time.

Where: Is it at a certain place?

Are you at a friend's house when you overeat? A mother-in-law's? In your own kitchen? Always at a party? Always in front of the TV?

What: Is it what you are feeling?

Are you feeling lonely, bored, or depressed when you overeat? Try to put a label on how you are feeling *before* you reach for food.

"Food, Mood, and Activity Record" and "Steps to Success" worksheets can be downloaded at www.1thingdiet.com.

Once we become aware of our eating triggers (or high-risk situations), our next step, of course, is coping with these high-risk situations.

CHAPTER 13:

Taming of the Shrew:
Making Those Necessary Changes

When patterns are broken, new worlds emerge.
~~Tuli Kupferberg

This is a follow up to identifying high-risk situations. Making necessary changes or coping with our high-risk situations is the next step.

Do you need to be extra cautious at a particular place from now on? Do you have to prepare ahead? Do you have trouble eating in moderation when you are with a particular person or group? Whatever you learned from the previous chapter, it is time to use this knowledge to your benefit.

The following questions are critical to answer in order to make necessary behavior changes:

What change(s) do you need to make to avoid an eating trigger(s):

1. _____
_____
_____

2. _____
    _____
    _____

How will you make such changes? (use "b" as your back-up plan)

1. a. _____
       _____
       _____

b. _____
    _____
    _____

2.a. _____
      _____
      _____

b. _____
    _____
    _____

Let's use Raymond (from the previous chapter) for one example. What change(s) do you need to make to avoid an eating trigger(s):

1. Be sure not to skip lunch. _____

How will you make such changes (use "b" as your back-up plan):

1. a. Pack a sandwich and fruit in A.M. so that I have a lunch handy to eat while working.
    b. (back up plan) Keep a healthy frozen meal or healthy canned soup at work for the day(s) I do not pack lunch.

If your trigger is due to a particular emotion, you might want to try the alternative activity method. There are many alternative activities to eating. What do you like to do (besides eat)? Do you like to dance? If you enjoy dancing, go in your bedroom or living room and turn on the music and dance, especially if you have an urge to eat. Do you like to walk? Take a brisk walk. This has many benefits, including the time it offers for you to think about what you are about to do: overeat. Do you like to nap? If your schedule allows, go take a nap. Did you know that many people overeat because they are tired? That's right, they think that food will give them more energy to stay awake. Also when you are tired, you care less about your caloric consumption that when you are rested.

List at least three things you thoroughly enjoy. (Do not be surprised if it takes a while to think of things):

———————————————————————————
———————————————————————————
———————————————————————————
———————————————————————————
———————————————————————————
———————————————————————————

These things you like to do for enjoyment are good "alternative activities" to eating or giving in to an eating trigger. If you enjoy it, you won't think they are a sacrifice or that they are "second fiddle" to eating.

Below is a list of alternative activities to eating:

Take a walk	Play a board game with your child or spouse
Call a friend	Dance to music
Visit a friend	Write a letter
Take a shower or bath	Work on a hobby
Chew sugar-free gum	Brush your teeth
Play with your dog or cat	Take a hike
Clean a room in the house	Ride a bike
Read a book	Make a scrapbook or look at old pictures
Take a nap	Imagine being fit (daydream!)

Hug your child	Do 5 minutes on the treadmill (or longer)
Go for a drive in car	Paint your fingernails (sorry, guys!)
Write in your food diary	Write in a journal
Go shopping for clothes	Pay the bills (forget it, this might be a trigger!)
Drink a large glass of water	

When you are deciding between giving in to your trigger or engaging in an alternative activity, please know that it is much easier to pick eating. The urge to eat is much stronger than the urge to do some of these things you enjoy. You have to consciously make the choice to pick the alternative activity. In time, the act of picking the alternative activity will become a learned behavior.

---

*Actual Story: Recently a patient of mine decided to do something about the stress she felt every day versus overeating when she felt this intense knot in her stomach. She decided to breathe deeply and visualize the knot in her stomach unclenching. In her own words, she "waited for the knot to clear" so she could "feel that she didn't need food."

By writing down what she ate in a food and mood diary, she was able to make the connection between her stress level and overeating. But then, she "tamed the shrew" by doing something about it.

This woman, who I think is very brave, lost 9 ½ pounds in 3 months. What I also think is so interesting about her story is that she told me, "I want to continue this. For once in my life, I don't feel like I have to diet." What a fantastic new attitude!

Trying to deal with the underlying feeling rather than turning to food is actually much harder. It is perhaps one of the most difficult things you may have to do. If you have tried several of the above techniques and still need help dealing with a particular emotion, you may want to seek professional therapy. Dealing with the emotion may take several visits with a therapist. You will be ahead of the game, however, in that you already have identified the feeling that is making your life harder than it has to be.

CHAPTER 14:

Keeping Your Nose to the Grindstone: Ongoing Motivation/Maintenance

When I throw my golf clubs, I'm sure to throw them in the direction that I'm playing.
~~President Ronald Reagan

Many of our great leaders or great minds know that setbacks are inevitable. It is how you handle the setbacks that really count. In other words, we may rant and rave and become emotional, but deep down we need to have faith in ourselves that we will get back on track. Many famous inventions were not thought of and developed on the first effort. Thomas Edison is the first who comes to mind when thinking about failures. He made many attempts to invent the efficient light bulb. What if he couldn't cope with his "failures?" His tenacity was the backbone to his success in a number of his accomplishments.

A relapse can be defined as a return to behavior which has previously stopped. Relapse prevention helps you identify the process of relapse and helps you develop coping skills to implement before your relapse process progresses to a full relapse of overeating and/or avoiding exercise.

I promised you that we would get back to David who lost 21 pounds, beginning with the breakdown of his car. David gained 3 pounds back rather quickly when he finally got his car repaired. Why? Because he returned to the behavior of driving places that he walked to previously. In order to manage this relapse, David had to find a way to build more activity into his daily routine to replace the walking. It took him a few weeks to develop a relapse plan of walking at the high school track near his apartment three times per week (not every day). He lost one of the 3 pounds he regained but then decided that was good enough. This, in my opinion, is a healthy reaction. *He is not going to be perfect and he is going to have a realistic expectation.*

In the last two chapters, we discussed (a) how to identify a high-risk situation and then (b) how to handle a high-risk situation. Handling a problematic situation in a healthy way is hard to do over time. It is inevitable that individuals will *not* continue to make good choices each time they are faced with a problem or situation that historically has given them trouble. Why? Because we are human beings. Some days we are more motivated than others. Some days we are more tired than others. Some days we see clearer than others. Some days we feel better about ourselves than other days, etc., etc., etc.

Sometimes our problematic situation could be an emotion or an unrealistic expectation. We may expect to make good decisions and healthy choices 100% of the time. If you are looking for perfection, you will never find it! If you are hoping to always be right, you won't be and you'll be terribly disappointed.

If you were taking the family on a road trip and took the wrong turn, would you say, "That's it, we've got to go home?" Then why give up on your effort to eating healthier and exercising more often? Turn your mistake into a valuable learning experience. What sights did you see along the way when you took the wrong turn? Did you have great conversation with your kids when on the wrong path in the car? Likewise, turn that "mistake" (I don't even like to use the word in weight management) of eating the cheesecake after dinner when you were out with friends into a learning experience: "Boy, I really loved that cake, but I guess I could have shared it with my two friends instead of eating the whole piece myself." Shake it off! Move forward! Tomorrow is not a new day, this moment is a new moment! Wipe the cake off of your face and move on.

How we respond to a setback separates "winners" from "losers." Realize that it is not a catastrophe that you had a piece of cheesecake. As soon as you think it is so negative that you had a dessert, you are more likely to make the situation worse and continue to overeat or eat high-fat or sweet foods.

My education has given me an opportunity to learn about addictions or problems other than food or weight management. An alcoholic once said to me, "It is not one thing after the other, it is the same thing time and time again." So while we can make every effort to identify a problem and cope in an improved way, sometimes there is an underlying issue to our bad behavior. If you have not identified a problem and found a better way to handle it (chapters 12 and 13), then you still have a lot of work to do. Likewise, if you have superficially identified the problem and handled it in a healthier way, you may still have a recurring, underlying problem that will get you into trouble time after time. For example, let's say you realize that getting angry leads you to overeating. You take a walk or use the treadmill to let off steam over and over again and this has been somewhat successful for avoiding a several-pound weight gain. Hats off to you! This is a wonderful step. What would really be the *best* solution to the recurring problem is to figure out why you get angry so often. Are your expectations of others too high? Are your expectations of yourself too high? Are you disappointed or angry with yourself? Who are you really angry at and why? Analyzing these types of questions may be beyond the scope of this book, but not handling an underlying issue takes on many forms in our behavior.

The other issue involved with maintaining a weight loss is your motivation level. In Chapter 5 we discussed listing the pros and cons of losing weight and then asking yourself how motivated you were on a scale of 1 to 10 (10 most motivated) to lose weight. Now the question might be: How motivated are you to *continue* to make efforts to lose weight or How motivated are you to *keep the weight off*. In any event, asking yourself is an important step. It's good to know where you stand with your level of motivation. What is your current motivational level (assuming you have already started to set out in your weight loss journey)? Write down the date and motivational level 1-10:

Date   Motivational Level

_____   1 2 3 4 5 6 7 8 9 10

Has it dropped or stayed the same since Chapter 5? If you are not motivated anymore, you need to ask yourself why. What's different about your attitude now than your attitude before?

A different attitude later usually involves having unrealistic expectations at the onset of your plans to lose weight. If you get discouraged because the weight loss was not great enough, you are sure to lose some degree of motivation. So, analyze how realistic your expectations were. This is why a whole chapter was designated to expectations. Remember Chapter 2, Get Real! The material in that chapter was emphasized to give you a good foundation so that disappointment did not set in and affect your attitude and, eventually, your motivation level.

Relapses happen more often when our degree of motivation wanes. If your motivational level has dropped and it is not due to unrealistic expectations, what is different about now versus before, when you first set out to lose weight? You may not know the answer off the top of your head. Take some time and really think about it. Has a situation in your life changed? Has your "hot button" (the reason you wanted to lose weight) changed?

Jot down your thoughts. My motivational level may have decreased because:

_____
_____
_____
_____
_____
_____

Whatever your reason is, do not give up. "Throw your golf clubs in the direction you are going anyway." No one accomplishes great things without being persistent. Take responsibility and pick "1 thing" to make you a little healthier today. Be patient, but persistent.

PART FIVE:

How's it Going? (Evaluation)

CHAPTER 15:

"1 Thing" Is A Lot!

Sometimes it's the smallest decisions that can change your life forever.
~~Keri Russell

We've covered a lot of ground together: Realistic expectations about weight loss, reasons for obesity and its relationship to diabetes and other health problems, readiness for behavior change, how calories are obtained and expended, basics of nutrition, importance of exercise and sleep in addition to good food, ideas to make food and activity changes in your life, how to become more aware of obesity-causing behaviors, what to do once you realize which behaviors are the culprit, and how to stay motivated! Wow!

Hopefully you have an understanding of each of these critical concepts. You do not have to be an expert at any of them, but having a conceptual idea of these components is a step in the right direction and, frankly, a foundation to lifelong weight management.

It is my sincere hope that you found some idea—whether an idea listed or your own creative idea—for a lifestyle change. Even if you lost 4 pounds while reading this book (hey, that will make the book sell!) or have lost 10 or 15 pounds after initiating some of the ideas or techniques, this is an accomplishment!

As we discussed in the previous chapters, you don't have to lose 40 pounds or get to your "ideal" body weight (a term we don't even use anymore), to keep diabetes or another lifestyle-causing health condition at bay. A five- or ten-pound loss has you that much closer to stopping the development of diabetes, for example. In fact, every pound lost pushes you a step back from developing an obesity-related health problem.

You can do this! You can make a necessary lifestyle change and make it very meaningful! Use the tools provided to you to analyze your daily regimen and make a change in your behavior. Write down the change and weigh yourself the day you make the change to see what effect the change has on your weight a few weeks or months later. Be patient. You are choosing *real* behavior change, not a diet this time. You have decided to use life skills rather than a diet book. Although this will be a bit more work than reading the diet book, you have given yourself a *gift*! –the gift of believing in yourself and your commitment to be healthy.

Go slowly; just pick one change. Don't be tempted to make more than one change unless you decide to make one diet and one activity change together, which is fine. Don't overwhelm yourself with too many changes at one time. That would be defeating the purpose here. Remember what happens when something becomes too difficult?

Re-read the book after some time has passed. This will help keep you motivated. Continue to ask yourself why you want to lose weight. It is OK if weeks go by and you are only maintaining your weight. Be patient and the weight loss will begin again. Slow and steady. If months go by and you are ready to add one more change, wonderful! This is *not* a race, but a journey.

Keep in touch during this journey. Write down your change and how it has affected your weight, your outlook, or anything else in your life. Write in to me at 1thingdiet.com. Best wishes for a healthy future!

References

Chapter 1: One Thing (Change) Means A Lot!
Augurs-Collins T, et al. A randomized controlled trial of weight reduction and exercise for diabetes management in older African-American subjects. *Diabetes Care* 1997; 20(10):1503-1511.

The Diabetes Control and Complications Trial Research Group (1993). The Effect of intensive treatment of diabetes on the development and progression of long-term complications in insulin-dependent diabetes mellitus. *N Engl J Med* 1993;329(14):977-986.

Wing R, et al. Long-term effects of modest weight loss in type II diabetic patients. *Arch Intern Med* 1987; 147:1749-1753.

Chapter 2: Get Real!
Savoye M, Berry D, Dziura, et al. Anthropometric and psychosocial changes in obese adolescents enrolled in a weight management program. *J Am Diet Assoc*. 2005; 105:364-370.

Chapter 3: Obesity: What is it? How did it get here?
Manson JE, et al Body weight and mortality among women. *N Engl J Med* 1995;333:677-685

Troiano R, et al The relationship between body weight and mortality: a quantitative analysis of combined information from existing studies. *Int J Obes* 1996;20;63-75.

Chapter 4: Diabetes: The Wrath of Obesity
American Diabetes Association. Standards of Medical Care in Diabetes 2011. *Diabetes Care* 2011 Jan; 34 Suppl 1:S11-61.

Shaw JE, Sicree RA, Zimmet PZ. Global estimates of the prevalence of diabetes for 2010 and 2030. *Diabetes Research and Clinical Practice* 2010; 87: 4-14.

Wild S, Roglic G, Green A, Sicree R, King H. Global prevalence of diabetes: estimates for the year 2000 and projections for 2030. *Diabetes Care* 2010; 27(5): 1047-1053.

Chapter 5: Are You Ready to Make Changes?
Brownell, KD. *The Learn Program for Weight Management*. American Health Publishing Company, Euless, TX, 2004.

Chapter 6: The Ins and Outs (calories in and out) of Weight Loss
Harrison Benedict Equation: http://www.bmi-calculator.net/bmr-calculator/harris-benedict-equation

Pennington J.A. and Spungen J. *Bowes and Church's Food Values of Portions Commonly Used*, Nineteenth Edition, J.B. Lippincott Company, Philadelphia, PA, 2010.

Chapter 7: Nutrition 101 and Donuts 540
Food and Nutrition Board, Institute of Medicine, National Academies. Dietary Reference Intakes (DRIs): Recommended Dietary Allowances and Adequate Intakes, Vitamins, 1998.

Food and Nutrition Board, Institute of Medicine, National Academies. Dietary Reference Intakes (DRIs): Recommended Dietary Allowances and Adequate Intakes, Elements, 1998.

Chapter 8: Get Up Off the Sofa!
Barry HC, Eathorne SW. Exercise and aging: Issues for practitioner. *Med Clin North Am* 1994; 78(2): 357-70.

Beere P, Russell S, Morey M, Kitzman D, Higginbotham M. Aerobic exercise training can reserve age-related peripheral circulatory changes in healthy older men. *Circulation* 1999; 100: 1085-1094.

Brownell, KD. *The Learn Program for Weight Management*. American Health Publishing Company, Euless, TX, 2004.

Chapter 9: Maybe You Should Count Sheep, Not Calories!

Itani O, Kaneita Y, Murata A, Yokoyama E, Onida T. Association of onset of obesity with sleep duration and shift work among Japanese adults. *Sleep Med* 2011, Mar 4 [Epub]

Inadequate sleep as a risk factor for obesity: analyses of NHANES 1. *Sleep* 2005; 10:1289-1296.

www.science.daily.com/releases/2006/07/06070312945.htm

Chapter 10: "1 Thing" Ideas: Making Better Food Choices

Pennington J.A. and Spungen J. *Bowes and Churchs Food Values of Portions Commonly Used*, Nineteenth Edition, J.B. Lippincott Company, Philadelphia, PA, 2010.

Chapter 11: "1 Thing" Ideas: Attaining More Activity

Nutristrategy.com

Chapter 12: Becoming More Aware

Savoye-DeSanti M and Barbetta G. *Smart Moves Weight Management Workbook*. www.smartmovesforkids.com

Chapter 13: Taming of the Shrew: Making those Necessary Changes

Savoye-DeSanti M and Barbetta G. *Smart Moves Weight Management Workbook*. www.smartmovesfordkids.com

Appendix A.1.

Dietary Reference Intakes (DRIs): Recommended Dietary Allowances and Adequate Intakes, Vitamins
Food and Nutrition Board, Institute of Medicine, National Academies

Life Stage Group	Vitamin A (µg/d)[a]	Vitamin C (mg/d)	Vitamin D (µg/d)[b,c]	Vitamin E (mg/d)[d]	Vitamin K (µg/d)	Thiamin (mg/d)	Riboflavin (mg/d)	Niacin (mg/d)[e]	Vitamin B6 (mg/d)	Folate (µg/d)[f]	Vitamin B12 (µg/d)	Pantothenic Acid (mg/d)	Biotin (µg/d)	Choline (mg/d)[g]
Infants														
0 to 6 mo	400*	40*	10	4*	2.0*	0.2*	0.3*	2*	0.1*	65*	0.4*	1.7*	5*	125*
6 to 12 mo	500*	50*	10	5*	2.5*	0.3*	0.4*	4*	0.3*	80*	0.5*	1.8*	6*	150*
Children														
1–3 y	**300**	**15**	**15**	**6**	30*	**0.5**	**0.5**	**6**	**0.5**	**150**	**0.9**	2*	8*	200*
4–8 y	**400**	**25**	**15**	**7**	55*	**0.6**	**0.6**	**8**	**0.6**	**200**	**1.2**	3*	12*	250*
Males														
9–13 y	**600**	**45**	**15**	**11**	60*	**0.9**	**0.9**	**12**	**1.0**	**300**	**1.8**	4*	20*	375*
14–18 y	**900**	**75**	**15**	**15**	75*	**1.2**	**1.3**	**16**	**1.3**	**400**	**2.4**	5*	25*	550*
19–30 y	**900**	**90**	**15**	**15**	120*	**1.2**	**1.3**	**16**	**1.3**	**400**	**2.4**	5*	30*	550*
31–50 y	**900**	**90**	**15**	**15**	120*	**1.2**	**1.3**	**16**	**1.3**	**400**	**2.4**	5*	30*	550*
51–70 y	**900**	**90**	**15**	**15**	120*	**1.2**	**1.3**	**16**	**1.7**	**400**	**2.4**[h]	5*	30*	550*
>70 y	**900**	**90**	**20**	**15**	120*	**1.2**	**1.3**	**16**	**1.7**	**400**	**2.4**[h]	5*	30*	550*
Females														
9–13 y	**600**	**45**	**15**	**11**	60*	**0.9**	**0.9**	**12**	**1.0**	**300**	**1.8**	4*	20*	375*
14–18 y	**700**	**65**	**15**	**15**	75*	**1.0**	**1.0**	**14**	**1.2**	**400**[i]	**2.4**	5*	25*	400*
19–30 y	**700**	**75**	**15**	**15**	90*	**1.1**	**1.1**	**14**	**1.3**	**400**[i]	**2.4**	5*	30*	425*
31–50 y	**700**	**75**	**15**	**15**	90*	**1.1**	**1.1**	**14**	**1.3**	**400**[i]	**2.4**	5*	30*	425*
51–70 y	**700**	**75**	**15**	**15**	90*	**1.1**	**1.1**	**14**	**1.5**	**400**	**2.4**[h]	5*	30*	425*
>70 y	**700**	**75**	**20**	**15**	90*	**1.1**	**1.1**	**14**	**1.5**	**400**	**2.4**[h]	5*	30*	425*
Pregnancy														
14–18 y	**750**	**80**	**15**	**15**	75*	**1.4**	**1.4**	**18**	**1.9**	**600**[j]	**2.6**	6*	30*	450*
19–30 y	**770**	**85**	**15**	**15**	90*	**1.4**	**1.4**	**18**	**1.9**	**600**[j]	**2.6**	6*	30*	450*
31–50 y	**770**	**85**	**15**	**15**	90*	**1.4**	**1.4**	**18**	**1.9**	**600**[j]	**2.6**	6*	30*	450*
Lactation														
14–18 y	**1,200**	**115**	**15**	**19**	75*	**1.4**	**1.6**	**17**	**2.0**	**500**	**2.8**	7*	35*	550*
19–30 y	**1,300**	**120**	**15**	**19**	90*	**1.4**	**1.6**	**17**	**2.0**	**500**	**2.8**	7*	35*	550*
31–50 y	**1,300**	**120**	**15**	**19**	90*	**1.4**	**1.6**	**17**	**2.0**	**500**	**2.8**	7*	35*	550*

NOTE: This table (taken from the DRI reports, see www.nap.edu) presents Recommended Dietary Allowances (RDAs) in **bold type** and Adequate Intakes (AIs) in ordinary type followed by an asterisk (*). An RDA is the average daily dietary intake level; sufficient to meet the nutrient requirements of nearly all (97-98 percent) healthy individuals in a group. It is calculated from an Estimated Average Requirement (EAR). If sufficient scientific evidence is not available to establish an EAR, and thus calculate an RDA, an AI is usually developed. For healthy breastfed infants, an AI is the mean intake. The AI for other life stage and gender groups is believed to cover the needs of all healthy individuals in the groups, but lack of data or uncertainty in the data prevent being able to specify with confidence the percentage of individuals covered by this intake.

[a] As retinol activity equivalents (RAEs). 1 RAE = 1 µg retinol, 12 µg β-carotene, 24 µg α-carotene, or 24 µg β-cryptoxanthin. The RAE for dietary provitamin A carotenoids is two-fold greater than retinol equivalents (RE), whereas the RAE for preformed vitamin A is the same as RE.

[b] As cholecalciferol. 1 µg cholecalciferol = 40 IU vitamin D.

[c] Under the assumption of minimal sunlight.

[d] As α-tocopherol. α-Tocopherol includes RRR-α-tocopherol, the only form of α-tocopherol that occurs naturally in foods, and the 2R-stereoisomeric forms of α-tocopherol (RRR-, RSR-, RRS-, and RSS-α-tocopherol) that occur in fortified foods and supplements. It does not include the 2S-stereoisomeric forms of α-tocopherol (SRR-, SSR-, SRS-, and SSS-α-tocopherol), also found in fortified foods and supplements.

[e] As niacin equivalents (NE). 1 mg of niacin = 60 mg of tryptophan; 0–6 months = preformed niacin (not NE).

[f] As dietary folate equivalents (DFE). 1 DFE = 1 µg food folate = 0.6 µg of folic acid from fortified food or as a supplement consumed with food = 0.5 µg of a supplement taken on an empty stomach.

[g] Although AIs have been set for choline, there are few data to assess whether a dietary supply of choline is needed at all stages of the life cycle, and it may be that the choline requirement can be met by endogenous synthesis at some of these stages.

[h] Because 10 to 30 percent of older people may malabsorb food-bound B12, it is advisable for those older than 50 years to meet their RDA mainly by consuming foods fortified with B12 or a supplement containing B12.

[i] In view of evidence linking folate intake with neural tube defects in the fetus, it is advisable for those older than 50 years to meet their RDA mainly by consuming foods fortified with B12 or a supplement containing B12. In view of evidence linking folate intake with neural tube defects in the fetus, it is recommended that all women capable of becoming pregnant consume 400 µg from supplements or fortified foods in addition to intake of food folate from a varied diet.

[j] It is assumed that women will continue consuming 400 µg from supplements or fortified food until their pregnancy is confirmed and they enter prenatal care, which ordinarily occurs after the end of the periconceptional period—the critical time for formation of the neural tube.

SOURCES: Dietary Reference Intakes for Calcium, Phosphorous, Magnesium, Vitamin D, and Fluoride (1997); Dietary Reference Intakes for Thiamin, Riboflavin, Niacin, Vitamin B6, Folate, Vitamin B12, Pantothenic Acid, Biotin, and Choline (1998); Dietary Reference Intakes for Vitamin C, Vitamin E, Selenium, and Carotenoids (2000); Dietary Reference Intakes for Vitamin A, Vitamin K, Arsenic, Boron, Chromium, Copper, Iodine, Iron, Manganese, Molybdenum, Nickel, Silicon, Vanadium, and Zinc (2001); Dietary Reference Intakes for Water, Potassium, Sodium, Chloride, and Sulfate (2005); and Dietary Reference Intakes for Calcium and Vitamin D (2011). These reports may be accessed via www.nap.edu.

Dietary Reference Intakes (DRIs): Recommended Dietary Allowances and Adequate Intakes, Elements
Food and Nutrition Board, Institute of Medicine, National Academies

Life Stage Group	Calcium (mg/d)	Chromium (µg/d)	Copper (µg/d)	Fluoride (mg/d)	Iodine (µg/d)	Iron (mg/d)	Magnesium (mg/d)	Manganese (mg/d)	Molybdenum (µg/d)	Phosphorus (mg/d)	Selenium (µg/d)	Zinc (mg/d)	Potassium (g/d)	Sodium (g/d)	Chloride (g/d)
Infants															
0 to 6 mo	200*	0.2*	200*	0.01*	110*	0.27*	30*	0.003*	2*	100*	15*	2*	0.4*	0.12*	0.18*
6 to 12 mo	260*	5.5*	220*	0.5*	130*	11	75*	0.6*	3*	275*	20*	3	0.7*	0.37*	0.57*
Children															
1–3 y	700	11*	340	0.7*	90	7	80	1.2*	17	460	20	3	3.0*	1.0*	1.5*
4–8 y	1,000	15*	440	1*	90	10	130	1.5*	22	500	30	5	3.8*	1.2*	1.9*
Males															
9–13 y	1,300	25*	700	2*	120	8	240	1.9*	34	1,250	40	8	4.5*	1.5*	2.3*
14–18 y	1,300	35*	890	3*	150	11	410	2.2*	43	1,250	55	11	4.7*	1.5*	2.3*
19–30 y	1,000	35*	900	4*	150	8	400	2.3*	45	700	55	11	4.7*	1.5*	2.3*
31–50 y	1,000	35*	900	4*	150	8	420	2.3*	45	700	55	11	4.7*	1.5*	2.3*
51–70 y	1,000	30*	900	4*	150	8	420	2.3*	45	700	55	11	4.7*	1.3*	2.0*
> 70 y	1,200	30*	900	4*	150	8	420	2.3*	45	700	55	11	4.7*	1.2*	1.8*
Females															
9–13 y	1,300	21*	700	2*	120	8	240	1.6*	34	1,250	40	8	4.5*	1.5*	2.3*
14–18 y	1,300	24*	890	3*	150	15	360	1.6*	43	1,250	55	9	4.7*	1.5*	2.3*
19–30 y	1,000	25*	900	3*	150	18	310	1.8*	45	700	55	8	4.7*	1.5*	2.3*
31–50 y	1,000	25*	900	3*	150	18	320	1.8*	45	700	55	8	4.7*	1.5*	2.3*
51–70 y	1,200	20*	900	3*	150	8	320	1.8*	45	700	55	8	4.7*	1.3*	2.0*
> 70 y	1,200	20*	900	3*	150	8	320	1.8*	45	700	55	8	4.7*	1.2*	1.8*
Pregnancy															
14–18 y	1,300	29*	1,000	3*	220	27	400	2.0*	50	1,250	60	12	4.7*	1.5*	2.3*
19–30 y	1,000	30*	1,000	3*	220	27	350	2.0*	50	700	60	11	4.7*	1.5*	2.3*
31–50 y	1,000	30*	1,000	3*	220	27	360	2.0*	50	700	60	11	4.7*	1.5*	2.3*
Lactation															
14–18 y	1,300	44*	1,300	3*	290	10	360	2.6*	50	1,250	70	13	5.1*	1.5*	2.3*
19–30 y	1,000	45*	1,300	3*	290	9	310	2.6*	50	700	70	12	5.1*	1.5*	2.3*
31–50 y	1,000	45*	1,300	3*	290	9	320	2.6*	50	700	70	12	5.1*	1.5*	2.3*

NOTE: This table (taken from the DRI reports, see www.nap.edu) presents Recommended Dietary Allowances (RDAs) in **bold type** and Adequate Intakes (AIs) in ordinary type followed by an asterisk (*). An RDA is the average daily dietary intake level; sufficient to meet the nutrient requirements of nearly all (97-98 percent) healthy individuals in a group. It is calculated from an Estimated Average Requirement (EAR). If sufficient scientific evidence is not available to establish an EAR, and thus calculate an RDA, an AI is usually developed. For healthy breastfed infants, an AI is the mean intake. The AI for other life stage and gender groups is believed to cover the needs of all healthy individuals in the groups, but lack of data or uncertainty in the data prevent being able to specify with confidence the percentage of individuals covered by this intake.

SOURCES: *Dietary Reference Intakes for Calcium, Phosphorous, Magnesium, Vitamin D, and Fluoride* (1997); *Dietary Reference Intakes for Thiamin, Riboflavin, Niacin, Vitamin B6, Folate, Vitamin B12, Pantothenic Acid, Biotin, and Choline* (1998); *Dietary Reference Intakes for Vitamin C, Vitamin E, Selenium, and Carotenoids* (2000); and *Dietary Reference Intakes for Vitamin A, Vitamin K, Arsenic, Boron, Chromium, Copper, Iodine, Iron, Manganese, Molybdenum, Nickel, Silicon, Vanadium, and Zinc* (2001); *Dietary Reference Intakes for Water, Potassium, Sodium, Chloride, and* **Sulfate** (2005); and *Dietary Reference Intakes for Calcium and Vitamin D* (2011). These reports may be accessed via www.nap.edu.

Appendix B.1. – Diet Change Record

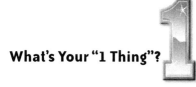

What's Your "1 Thing"?

I will make the following *diet change* each day:

This change will happen <u>one time, two times, three times</u> (circle one) per day. This will save me _____ calories per day. This will help me lose _____ pounds per month/year.

Do calculation:

Weight before the change _____ Date _____

Wk/Mo	Date	Weight	Comments
1			
2			
3			
4			
5			
6			
7			
8			
9			
10			
11			
12			

13			
14			
15			
16			
17			
18			
19			
20			
21			
22			
23			
24			
25			
26			
27			
28			
29			
30			
31			
32			
33			
34			
35			

36			
37			
38			
39			
40			
41			
42			
43			
44			
45			
46			
47			
48			
49			
50			
51			
52			
Total Lost			

Appendix B.2. – Activity Change Record

What's Your "1Thing"?

I will make the following *activity change* each day:

_____

This change will happen <u>one time, two times, three times</u> (circle one) per day.
This will burn _____ calories per day. This will help me lose _____
pounds per month/year.

Do calculation:

Weight before the change _____ **Date** _____

Wk/Mo	Date	Weight	Comments*
1			
2			
3			
4			
5			
6			
7			
8			
9			
10			
11			

12			
13			
14			
15			
16			
17			
18			
19			
20			
21			
22			
23			
24			
25			
26			
27			
28			
29			
30			
31			
32			
33			
34			

35			
36			
37			
38			
39			
40			
41			
42			
43			
44			
45			
46			
47			
48			
49			
50			
51			
52			
Total Lost			

*May want to keep track of percentage of body fat in this column. This should be obtained monthly using a body fat analyzer. When we increase activity, our muscle mass increases while fat mass decreases. Muscle weighs more than fat so this progress may not be evident if obtaining only weight on a regular basis.

Appendix B.3. –
Diet and Activity Change Record

What's Your "1Thing"?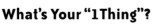

I will make one *diet and activity change* each day: (List each)

_____

_____

The diet change will happen <u>one time, two times, three times</u> (circle one) per day. This will save me _____ calories per day.

The activity change will happen <u>one time, two times, three times</u> (circle one) per day. This will burn an additional _____ calories per day.

The diet and activity change, together, will help me lose _____ pounds per month/year.

Do calculations:

Weight before diet and activity change _____ Date _____

Wk/Mo	Date	Weight	Comments*
1			
2			
3			
4			
5			
6			

7			
8			
9			
10			
11			
12			
13			
14			
15			
16			
17			
18			
19			
20			
21			
22			
23			
24			
25			
26			
27			
28			
29			

30			
31			
32			
33			
34			
35			
36			
37			
38			
39			
40			
41			
42			
43			
44			
45			
46			
47			
48			
49			
50			
51			
52			

Total Lost			

*May want to keep track of percentage body fat in this column. This should be obtained monthly using a body fat analyzer. When we increase activity, our muscle mass increases while fat mass decreases. Muscle weighs more than fat so this progress may not be evident if obtaining only weight on a regular basis.

CPSIA information can be obtained at www.ICGtesting.com
Printed in the USA
BVOW080713240512

290907BV00002B/1/P